THE NIGHTINGALE 6

Frameworks with Guidelines to Reduce Nurse Staffing Shortages

Gary Bruno BSN, CMSRN, GERO-BC, OCN

EAT THE ELEPHANT PUBLISHING

Edited By: Sabo Ace and Claire Harris

THE NIGHTINGALE 6: Frameworks with Guidelines to Reduce Nurse Staffing Shortages

Contributions

Editors: Sabo Ace & Claire Harris

Cover Design: Farrukh Khan

Interior Layout Design: Isa Reader @ luminousproject

Infographics Designer and Rendition: Lisa @pixelscreative from Fivver

Line/Copy Editor, Proofreader: Sabo Ace

Developmental Editor: Claire Harris

Infographic Original Concepts: Gary Bruno RN-BC

DEDICATION

To my late mother Marie Mimose Bruno, watching you struggle with the complications from diabetes and kidney failure remains a driving force for the care I provide each and every time I am on a unit.

You are truly missed.

PROFESSIONAL ACKNOWLEDGEMENTS

PROFESSIONAL ACKNOWLEDGEMENTS

I would like to thank the following individuals for using their time, experience and clinical expertise on providing feedback and peer review on the frameworks and guidelines that encompass this book. Your efforts are much appreciated.

Heather Mae Royer, BSN, MSN

9 years Nurse Manager experience, 24 total years in Nursing

Ryan Moar, BSN, MS, MBA, CCRN, CBRN

9 years Nurse Manager experience, 19 total years in Nursing

Karen M. Carpenter (Retired)

8 years Clinical Resource Nurse Educator experience, 44 total years in Nursing

Megan Malloy, RN, CCRN, PCCN, TCRN

3 years Clinical Resource Nurse Educator experience, 9 total years in Nursing

Kimberly LaRock, BSN, PCCN

1 Year Clinical Resource Nurse Educator experience, 9 total years in Nursing

CONTENTS

A BEDSIDE STORY

THE NIGHTINGALE 6

A BEDSIDE STORY

Even before getting report from the overnight nurse, Marie knew the day ahead would be a nightmare. The nurse manager had worked overnight because the unit was so short-staffed. That was never a good sign.

With a tight knot forming in her stomach, she braced herself for the chaos that always seemed to follow in the manager's wake and agreed to pick up yet another shift, making it her fifth 12-hour shift in a row. The fatigue had already set in, and anxiety was starting to wear on her nerves.

"I need you to orient Judith. We had two call-ins... sorry about that," the manager said, her apology as flat as the forced smile she wore.

Marie, a Nurse Liaison Mentor and veteran nurse with nine years of experience, was widely regarded as a clinical resource and trusted teammate. Normally, she would take the lead in orienting new nurses, but today their combined assignment involved caring for seven patients. The ideal patient-to-nurse ratio for the unit was 1:5.

"So, you want me to orient Judith, who's already had four different preceptors, and still take on patients? I have no idea where she even is in her training," Marie shot back. The frustration and concern in her voice caught the attention of other RNs nearby. As they gave and received shift reports, several exchanged looks of shared apprehension.

"Yes," replied the overnight charge nurse. "Judith can take four patients. Unfortunately, staffing doesn't have anyone available who can manage our cardiac drips. The day supervisor is tied up with numbers on another unit. The other two nurses already have eight patients each, so the day charge will handle four patients plus the open bed. I'm really sorry. Last night was brutal. I still haven't charted on two of my patients."

As she made her way to an empty computer desk with Judith, Marie couldn't help but think how nice it would be to have an office job. One where her nursing license wouldn't be on the line every week.

Once report was completed, the assignment was divided. Judith took four patients, and Marie took two. Marie set expectations for micro-huddles during the first four hours of the shift to help Judith stay on track with medication administration and patient assessments.

One of Judith's patients in Room 56 had a blood pressure that was lower than normal and had been steadily decreasing with each set of overnight vitals. Concerned, they decided to assess the patient together.

The patient was lethargic but easily aroused, reported no pain, and had a significant cardiac history, which was why she was on a cardiac monitor. After completing a head-to-toe assessment and obtaining vital signs, they noted the blood pressure remained slightly low. However, the patient was still receiving a fluid bolus, started by the overnight nurse to stabilize her pressure. They agreed to repeat a set of vitals once the bolus finished to determine its effectiveness.

With only one Patient Care Technician available to assist the entire unit, Judith offered to head back to Room 56 and get the next set of vitals.

An hour later, both Judith and Marie were swallowed up helping the other two overwhelmed nurses manage their patient loads. During that time, the cardiac monitor for Room 56 began alarming. The patient's heart rate slipped from 55 beats per minute to 50, then to 40.

Alarm fatigue, an all-too-common issue on nursing units, combined with the strain of being stretched too thin, delayed a prompt response to the alerts.

When Judith finally noticed the flashing telemetry monitor and hurried into Room 56, she found the patient difficult to wake, pale, and clammy. A fresh set of vitals showed a blood pressure of 60/40. Panic set in. Judith had never handled a patient this critical before. Without hesitation, she bolted from the room to find Marie.

They rushed in together and immediately saw the heart rate dipping into the 30s. Marie hit the emergency response button and took command of the room, calmly but urgently directing Judith through the necessary steps to stabilize the patient. Within minutes, the Code team and house supervisor arrived. Over the next 35 minutes, the team worked relentlessly, performing compressions, intubation, and administering emergency medications until the patient was finally stabilized.

Preparations began to transfer her to the Medical Intensive Care Unit.

By 10:05 a.m., the full weight of the morning was crashing down on Marie. Of the four patients assigned to them, only two had been seen, assessed, and medicated. The remaining two were waiting, with more than fifty medications queued up to be given. Daily care tasks such as baths, ambulation, and wound care were still undone. The unit was chaos. Discharges, new admissions, phone calls. The code documentation wasn't even charted yet, and Marie still had to debrief Judith before the shift ended.

The stress crept up in her chest like a heavy knot. The endless, mounting list of tasks felt like a wave threatening to drown her. She took a deep breath, trying to gather herself. But the truth was clear: the nightmare was fully underway, and there was no way out.

Moments later, the house supervisor stormed over, telemetry printouts in hand, her face flushed and her tone sharp.

"So, you two left your patient bradycardic for almost an hour and did nothing?"

Judith, already emotionally wrecked from the morning, couldn't manage a response. Tears filled her eyes as she turned away and quietly left, her shoulders heavy under the weight of the accusation.

Marie stood her ground. Her mind raced, her pulse pounded, but she remained still. She nodded—not in agreement with the tone of the accusation, but as a quiet acknowledgment that this moment, right here, was the breaking point.

She opened her mouth to explain how staffing shortages had led to this. How the situation wasn't the fault of any one person. But her thoughts drifted. She imagined an office job. A quiet, steady desk. A guaranteed lunch break. A job where her nursing license wasn't at constant risk.

The image was so vivid, so inviting, it almost felt like a lifeline.

This was it.

The final straw.

Marie knew, with a clarity that surprised her, that she would resign. She would leave the bedside for good. The relief that thought brought was a strange companion to her sorrow. But it was time. The floor had taken too much from her.

Since 1976, Americans have been asked which profession they trust most. Since nurses were first added to that poll in 1999, they have ranked number one for honesty and ethics every year except for one—in 2001, when firefighters briefly held the top spot after 9/11 (Saad, 2025).

That level of trust is extraordinary, especially when you consider what the profession is up against: an aging workforce on the verge of retirement, a critical gap in clinical experience for the generation of younger nurses, and a wave of job dissatisfaction driven by compassion fatigue, burnout, and impossible patient ratios.

Being ranked number one is a testament to the daily influence nurses have on patients and the vital role they play in the healthcare system. But the story you just read isn't rare. It is becoming routine.

The true stories in this book shine a light on what nurses are facing every day, illustrating the real-world consequences of an overburdened, understaffed, and increasingly fragile profession.

This isn't just a collection of stories. It is a call to action. These guidelines and frameworks were written for those ready to be part of the solution.

For the veteran nurse, nearing retirement but still eager to leave a mark on the profession.

For the new nurse, approaching the one-year mark after licensure and already wondering if this career is sustainable.

For the nurse manager, desperate for tools to turn around a disengaged, high-turnover unit.

If you're ready to be a change agent, this book is for you. Staffing shortages are a crisis. But with the right tools, strategies, and people willing to fight for the profession, we can begin to turn the tide.

SHORTAGES: IMPACTS AND SOLUTIONS

SHORTAGES: IMPACTS AND SOLUTIONS

Staffing shortages have always been woven into the history of nursing. Back in 1900, there were about 600 hospital-based nursing schools in the U.S., operating under what would now be called an apprenticeship model (Lynaugh, 1989). Students learned on the job, performing procedures specific to each hospital's standards. In exchange for education and a modest stipend, student nurses provided the bulk of patient care (Reverby, 1987).

But the truth was harsher than the advertisements. These schools were built more to meet staffing demands than to provide a quality education. It was an exploitative system. Young women worked 12-hour days, six days a week, fifty weeks a year, in strict, paternalistic conditions. When their training ended, there was no guarantee of employment. In fact, many hospitals refused to hire their own graduates (West, 2014). At the time, nursing was still viewed as a vocational trade and had not yet transitioned into a professional career with a deeper academic foundation and licensure requirements. As a result, by 1920, nearly 80 percent of nurses worked independently as private duty caregivers (Goldmark, 1984).

This private duty model had its own challenges. Nurses formed agreements and worked directly with patients and families, assuming full responsibility for care in the home. However, not everyone could afford private services after hospitalization. Students in training facilities provided most inpatient care for low-income patients, while those working privately faced income instability. Cases were scattered, transportation to remote towns was difficult, and few families could consistently pay for private care.

Private nursing services placed a financial burden on families yet still failed to provide nurses with reliable, livable wages (Burgess, 1984). Between 1900 and 1920, the two main sources of nursing labor—hospital training schools and private duty work—were at the heart of nationwide shortages.

During the Great Depression, conditions worsened. Hospitals and private practices slashed staff in order to survive financially. Thousands of nurses became unemployed, with too few opportunities to meet growing healthcare needs.

By the 1930s, the private care model began to collapse. Middle-class families who could no longer afford private duty nurses demanded more personalized care in hospitals. At the same time, facilities were transitioning away from multi-bed single ward model and moving toward private and semi-private rooms, which increased the demand for professional nursing staff. In response, hospitals redistributed responsibilities among graduates, students, and nurse aides. Healthcare leaders began to view private duty nursing as outdated and inefficient (Falk et al., 1933).

By the end of the Depression, staff nursing positions became the primary form of employment. In 1935, mandatory licensure for nurses was passed, though it was not fully enforced until after World War II. Titles such as Registered Nurse (RN) and Licensed Practical Nurse (LPN) became legally protected in all states (Egenes, n.d.).

By 1941, institutional nurses—often referred to as general staff nurses—made up 47 percent of active registered nurses. Private duty nurses accounted for 27 percent (McIver, 1942). However, transitioning from independent contractor roles to hospital employment was not easy. Many nurses resisted, holding onto their autonomy, especially as hospitals continued to treat them as low-cost labor. It wasn't until after World War II that hospitals began focusing on recruiting and retaining licensed staff nurses for bedside care.

Even then, resistance persisted. The institutional control of hospitals, paired with minimal nurse input, led to renewed waves of dissatisfaction and a return of staffing shortages.

The situation became so serious that, in 1947, the U.S. Department of Labor commissioned a national study to investigate the root causes of the crisis. *The Economic Status of Registered Professional Nurses 1946–47* was a 69-page report that exposed a profession burdened by low wages, harsh working conditions, and a desperate need for recognition and support. Among its most important findings were:

Wages and Salaries

In 1946–47, nurses' salaries remained low compared to those of other professions requiring similar education and training. Pay varied depending on the type of facility, geographical location, and level of experience. Most nurses worked in hospitals, where wages were typically lower than in private duty or specialized care settings.

Working Conditions

Nurses regularly endured long hours, with shifts often stretching far beyond the standard 40-hour workweek. This was especially true in hospitals, where chronic understaffing forced nurses to cover multiple shifts without adequate rest. The report highlighted both the physical and emotional toll the profession took on its practitioners.

Education and Training

At the time, most nurses received their education through hospital-based programs that combined practical experience with limited theoretical instruction. However, a growing push for standardized, formal nursing education was gaining momentum. The aim was to improve both patient care quality and professional competency.

Professionalization and Status

In 1946–47, nursing was still fighting for recognition as a fully respected profession. Nurses were largely viewed as subordinates to physicians, with minimal opportunities for career advancement or professional autonomy. Early efforts were underway to elevate the status of nursing through education reform and the formation of professional organizations that advocated for the field.

Labor Unionization

The post-war era saw a noticeable rise in labor union activity among nurses. Driven by demands for better wages, improved working conditions, and a greater voice in healthcare policy, more nurses began joining unions. Although unionization was still in its early stages, it marked a critical step toward collective advocacy in the profession (United States Department of Labor, 1948).

Ongoing Challenges and Institutional Resistance

Despite comprehensive studies like *The Economic Status of Registered Professional Nurses 1946–47*, hospitals remained reluctant to address nurses' concerns. Problems such as poor working conditions, disorganized wards, verbal abuse from both providers and patients, and a lack of professional recognition persisted. Rather than implement meaningful reforms, hospitals often hired temporary substitutes or aggressively recruited new nurses into the profession without addressing underlying issues.

Advocacy and Legislative Progress

Much of the foundational progress in nursing came through the persistent efforts of professional associations advocating for legal protections and standardized practices. In 1902, members of the newly formed New York Nurses Association convened at Rochester City Hospital to discuss the establishment of the nation's first Nurse Practice Act. In a historic moment, an elderly and frail Susan B. Anthony attended the meeting and urged the group to recognize the power and influence of their work (Willis et al., 2013).

Between 1940 and 1980, approximately 14 states passed or amended their Nurse Practice Acts to more clearly define nursing roles, responsibilities, and scope of practice. These legislative milestones reflected both the increasing complexity of healthcare delivery and the growing professional identity of the nursing field.

Evolution of Care Delivery Models

As demands on healthcare systems grew, hospitals were forced to reevaluate their staffing structures. By the 1960s and 1970s, a modern three-tiered nursing care delivery model emerged. This system included Registered Nurses (RNs), Licensed Practical Nurses (LPNs), and Unlicensed Assistive Personnel (UAPs), such as Patient Care Technicians. Despite these structural changes, nurses had little influence on how the model was developed. They continued to bear responsibility for the majority of direct patient care in hospitals, a dynamic that still exists today.

Modern Day Shortages

Staffing shortages in today's nursing units arise from several interconnected factors. Surveys consistently show that nurses cite toxic work environments, burnout, overwhelming workloads, and poor unit management as the leading reasons for leaving their positions.

Toxic Work Environment

A toxic work environment refers to a culture where negative behaviors—such as infighting, gossip, manipulation, bullying, and intimidation—become normalized. These behaviors can become ingrained over time, undermining productivity, eroding trust, and increasing stress. In healthcare, such environments are particularly harmful. The issue often begins long before nurses enter the workforce and continues throughout their careers.

A significant portion of nurses leave their first job because of the behavior of coworkers. Bullying, in particular, contributes to the worsening nurse shortage. A toxic culture leads to lower patient satisfaction, higher turnover rates, and negative outcomes in patient safety (Edmonson & Zelonka, 2019).

These environments often develop gradually, as harmful behaviors go unchecked. Leadership and colleagues may tolerate or even excuse such behavior as a coping mechanism in high-stress settings. The toll this takes on nurses' mental health is substantial, and one of the most common consequences is burnout.

Burnout

Burnout is characterized by physical and emotional exhaustion, along with a loss of motivation. It is typically caused by prolonged stress or frustration and impacts not only nurses' personal well-being but also their interactions with patients and the organizations they serve. Behavioral signs of burnout include isolation, poor judgment, and procrastination.

Emotionally, burnout may show up as reduced patient engagement and noticeable changes in bedside manner. Nurses experiencing burnout often exhibit a lack of empathy, decreased compassion, and rising cynicism. These signs are frequently seen in once-vibrant nurses who begin to seem less patient, less helpful, or even withdrawn and irritable with patients. This disengagement reduces productivity and increases absenteeism. As a result, the burden of care shifts to other nurses on the unit, fueling a cycle of stress and disengagement that affects the entire team.

Greater Workloads

The term *nursing workload* is frequently used in healthcare, but it often lacks a precise definition. Workload refers to the time and energy a nurse must devote to their responsibilities, including both direct and indirect patient care. A more modern understanding also includes time spent on workplace obligations and professional development (Alghamdi, 2016).

Nursing workload typically falls into two categories: direct patient care and non-patient care. Both are essential and must be completed during a nurse's shift, regardless of how busy the day becomes.

Non-patient care includes documentation, communication (such as emails or updates via platforms like Haiku), completion of required educational modules, and coordination with family members, providers, and interdisciplinary teams on patient care plans and clinical updates.

Direct patient care involves physically assessing patients, administering medications and other physician-ordered treatments, and delivering bedside care. Nurses are also expected to evaluate the effectiveness of interventions, adjust plans accordingly, and communicate changes to covering providers.

As nurse-to-patient ratios increase, these responsibilities become harder to manage. Each additional patient stretches the nurse thinner and reduces their ability to deliver effective, timely care. This increases the likelihood of poor patient outcomes.

Poor Unit Management

A significant portion of this book is devoted to exploring the role of the Nurse Manager. A detailed breakdown of responsibilities and guidelines for improving unit management can be found in Part 5 of *Nightingale 6*.

Units led by engaged, effective Nurse Managers typically experience lower turnover and fewer staffing shortages. These leaders actively invest in their teams, promote collaboration, and cultivate an environment that encourages growth, trust, and shared accountability.

On the other hand, poor unit management plays a central role in creating toxic workplace cultures. When Nurse Managers fail to support their teams, neglect opportunities for staff development, or dismiss the importance of collaboration, it often leads to high turnover and a dysfunctional work environment.

The Negative Costs

NSI is a national healthcare retention and nurse staffing firm that publishes an in-depth annual report on the current state of hospital nurse staffing. The 2024 report uses survey data from 400 hospitals across 36 states. In total, it reflects input from 723,691 healthcare workers, including 194,111 Registered Nurses (RNs).

Key findings from the 2024 report include:

1. The average cost of turnover for a bedside RN is $56,300, with a range between $45,100 and $67,500. For the average hospital, this results in a financial loss of $3.9 million to $5.8 million per year, per services. Each percentage point change in nurse staffing turnover equates to a $262,500 gain or loss per year.
2. The national RN vacancy rate remains high at 9.9 percent.
3. The RN Recruitment Difficulty Index averages 86 days. It takes nearly three months to recruit an experienced RN, with Medical-Surgical units facing the greatest challenges.
4. Nurses in step-down, telemetry, and emergency departments have been the most mobile, with cumulative four-year turnover rates of 119.0 percent, 115.9 percent, and 112.1 percent, respectively. This means that these services are turning over a units worth of nursing staff every year.

For better context, let's say a nursing service line has four units, with a combined 160 nurses. A 100% four-year turnover rate means that service is losing an average of 40 nurses per year over the course of four years. These losses are often supplemented with the use of travel nurses.

Currently, it is not uncommon to find nursing units that are 20% to 50% staffed by travel nurses.

5. About 30.2 percent of all new hires left within one year. This group also accounted for 40.4 percent of all turnovers. Additionally, 62.2 percent of nurses who exited had less than two years of service (NSI, 2024).

The financial burden is only part of the story. Since 2020, nurses have been retiring at an accelerated pace. Currently, 55 percent of nurses are over the age of 55, an estimated <u>one million nurses</u> plan to retire within the next decade. To compound the problem, the youngest members of the baby boomer generation will become eligible for retirement starting in 2030.

THE NURSING DOOM LOOP

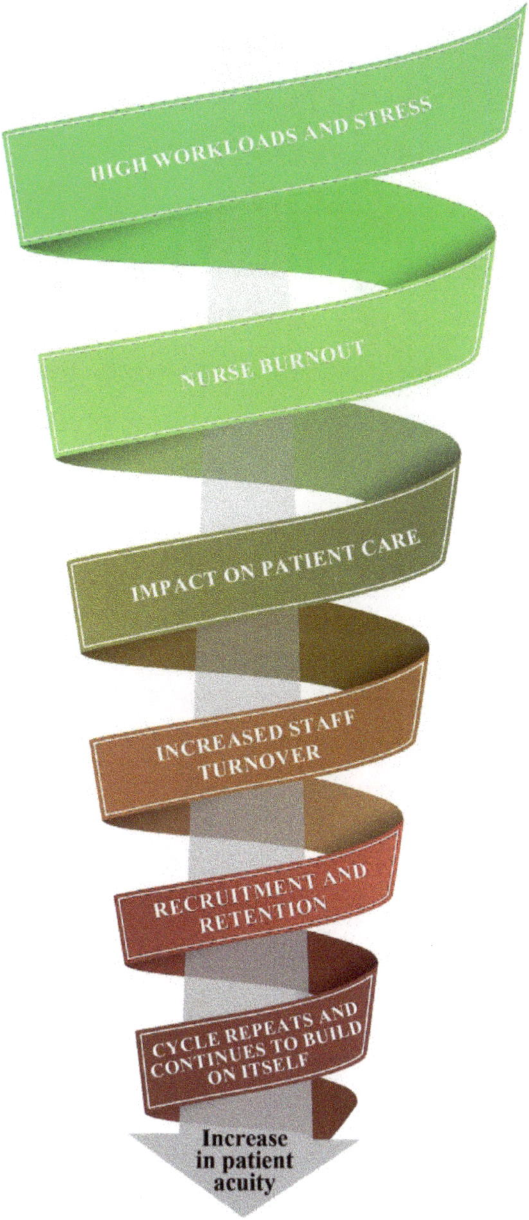

The Nursing Doom Loop is a self-perpetuating cycle that drives ongoing staffing shortages in hospitals, especially in nursing units. This cycle negatively affects both patient care and staff well-being, and once it begins, it becomes increasingly difficult to break.

1. High Workloads and Stress

- *Lack of Cohesion*: Many nursing units lack clear frameworks for building team cohesion.
- *Ineffective Teamwork*: Without strong teamwork, workloads increase. This leads to physical and emotional exhaustion, burnout, and elevated stress among nurses.

2. Nurse Burnout

- *Excessive Stress*: Over time, toxic behaviors and incivility become normalized within the work culture, contributing to widespread burnout.
- *Impact of Burnout*: Burnt-out nurses are more likely to take sick leave, resign, or exit the profession entirely.
- *Increased Patient Acuity*: As patient acuity increases, so does the demand on nurses.
- *Definition of Patient Acuity*: Patient acuity refers to the level of care a patient requires, based on the complexity of their condition and the intensity of nursing interventions (Habasevich, 2012). Higher acuity demands more time, skill, and resources.

3. Decreased Job Satisfaction

- *Dissatisfaction*: As stress and burnout worsen, job satisfaction declines. Nurses often leave in search of less demanding roles with better support and teamwork.

4. Increased Staff Turnover

- *Higher Turnover Rates*: Burnout and dissatisfaction lead to elevated turnover.
- *Impact of Inexperienced Staff*: As experienced nurses leave, hospitals hire and train new staff. These less experienced nurses often struggle to handle the workload, which creates additional strain.
- *The Vicious Cycle*: Hospitals enter a loop of constant hiring, training, and losing staff. This pattern continues to drive staffing shortages.

5. Recruitment and Retention Challenges

- *Poor Unit Management*: Units with poor leadership develop reputations that deter new candidates.
- *Retention Struggles*: Retaining veteran nurses becomes increasingly difficult due to rising retirements and unmanageable workloads.
- *Reinforcing the Cycle*: Inadequate staffing increases stress on the remaining nurses, leading to even more departures and furthering the cycle.

6. Impact on Patient Care

- *Stretched Nurses*: With fewer staff available, nurses are overwhelmed and unable to deliver timely, high-quality care.
- *Negative Outcomes*: High patient-to-nurse ratios contribute to medical errors, higher mortality rates, and lower patient satisfaction.
- *Impact on Morale*: These outcomes further damage team morale and increase emotional exhaustion.
- *Reinforcement of the Doom cycle*: Without strategic, team-based solutions to improve culture and operations, the cycle continues. The result is a workforce in decline and patient care that suffers.

HOW TO USE THIS BOOK

- *The Nightingale 6* provides clear, actionable guidelines organized around six core frameworks. These are designed to help move a nursing unit from survival mode to a more empowered, thriving state. Each framework offers practical, implementable steps to transform workplace culture, strengthen teamwork, and improve patient care outcomes.

The six frameworks are:

- *Shifting the Culture*
- *Creating and Utilizing Unit Councils*
- *Enhancing Coaching (Precepting)*
- *Maintaining Commitment*

- *Increasing a Unit's Capabilities*
- *Implementing Continuity*
- Each of these frameworks contains specific strategies that can lead to meaningful change within a nursing unit. The book is divided into two parts:
- Frameworks 1 to 3 are intended for nurses working on the front lines. These chapters provide tools to help nurses take ownership of their work environment and embrace the role of change agents. The goal is to shift attention from persistent challenges toward collaboration and solutions.
- Frameworks 4 to 6 are designed for leadership teams – including Educators, Clinical Leaders, and Nurse Managers. These sections address the reality that many leaders are placed in high-stakes roles without adequate resources or formal leadership training. These chapters offer structured guidance to help leaders shape, influence, and sustain effective change within their teams. This book is intended to be a resource. As a resource it will be something you will read through and then keep in your tool box, coming back to it again and again. Why? As Einstein said, never memorize anything you can look up.

WHY CHANGE IS HARD

Change is difficult because the human brain is biologically wired to seek comfort in routine and familiarity. When faced with something new, it's natural to feel uncertain, apprehensive, or even resistant. These instincts can cause individuals — and entire units — to remain stuck in ineffective or outdated patterns, even when those patterns are no longer serving them.

For nurses, operating in difficult gray areas is often part of the job. It is hard to manage a six- to eight-patient assignment when there is only one patient care technician available. It is hard to work alongside toxic coworkers who avoid responsibility, ignore call lights, and undermine morale. It is hard, as a manager, to open yet another resignation letter and wonder how the remaining team will cope.

Yet, nurses are the backbone of the healthcare system. In the United States, there are approximately 4.7 million nurses, and 89 percent of them work in direct patient care roles (AACN, 2024). Nurses serve as the critical link between patients and the broader healthcare team. They are often the ones coordinating care, advocating for patients, and filling communication gaps to keep care delivery cohesive and centered on patient needs.

This work is undeniably difficult. But with the right tools, a shift in approach, and the determination to do things differently, it is possible to lighten that burden. Not by working harder or doing more, but by changing how we engage with the challenges we face.

Rest assured, these frameworks have been used individually and in combination in multiple units and hospitals. Despite the initial struggles with implementation, over a period of time with consistency and supportive focus, the units who utilized these solutions made great leaps forward in reducing their staffing shortages.

The First Framework: Shifting the Culture

The first of the six frameworks focuses on what is arguably the most essential component of any nursing unit: its culture. A unit's culture sets the tone for everything else — how the team communicates, how challenges are approached, and how resilience is either nurtured or neglected.

A healthy culture builds stronger, more engaged teams. It supports empowerment, collaboration, and adaptability. More importantly, it becomes the foundation upon which all other improvements can be built. Culture is where sustainable change begins. It is also where the weight of nursing can begin to feel just a little lighter.

N1

SHIFTING CULTURE

"The Standard is the Standard."
— Mike Tomlin

N1
SHIFTING CULTURE

Theresa was a newly graduated nurse on a fast-paced medical-surgical unit. For the past two years, she had worked there as a Patient Care Technician and believed she had built strong relationships with her team. Her colleagues often praised her dedication, and several even wrote glowing recommendations for her nursing school application. They invited her to after-work gatherings, cheered her on during school, and encouraged her to return to the unit after earning her degree.

To Theresa, this place felt like home — a space where she was valued, supported, and part of something meaningful.

But stepping into her new role as a nurse, she quickly discovered that being a nurse was a very different experience from being a tech. The unit that had once felt like family began to challenge her in ways she never expected.

The shift in atmosphere was immediate. It felt like she had entered a different workplace — colder and more rigid. The same nurses who had once rooted for her now barely acknowledged her, especially when she made mistakes common to any new graduate. Her preceptor frequently reprimanded her in front of patients, leaving her embarrassed and humiliated.

When Theresa asked questions during report, the outgoing nurse would sigh, roll her eyes, and say, "Ask your preceptor," before walking away.

But the most painful moments came when she overheard her coworkers making disparaging remarks as she passed by the enclosed medication room. These were the same people she had once admired and trusted. Hearing their words stung in a way no formal reprimand could. It left her questioning not just her skills, but whether she still belonged in the place she once considered home.

Four months after finishing orientation, Theresa was assigned to float to another medical-surgical unit. As she stepped onto the new floor, she approached the unit secretary's desk, unsure of what kind of welcome she would receive.

The secretary greeted her with a warm smile. "You must be our float. Welcome to the 8200 Unit. Here are the passcodes for the locked doors and medication room."

Theresa was pleasantly surprised. She was used to scrambling for access codes — often having to chase down staff who would jot them on sticky notes she discarded by the end of her shift. This small, thoughtful gesture felt like a breath of fresh air.

Before she could settle in, the Charge Nurse approached with a stack of papers in hand.

"I'm sorry to throw this at you right away," she said kindly. "The other nurse had to leave for a family emergency. Here's the written report. Once you're ready, we can check the rooms together to make sure all the patients are safe."

As the shift progressed, Theresa's anxiety began to ease. She noticed subtle but powerful differences in how this unit functioned. Unlike other medical-surgical floors she had worked on, this team had practices in place that made the work feel less chaotic and more intentional. There was a calmness in how they moved and a kindness in how they spoke to one another.

For the first time in a long while, Theresa felt a flicker of hope.

Maybe things could be different.

Three cultural qualities stood out to her:

1. Clear Expectations

During team huddles and shift handoffs, expectations were clearly communicated and consistently reinforced. Visual reminders throughout the unit helped the team stay aligned and focused on shared goals.

2. Patient-Centered Teamwork

The team operated with a unified commitment to patient care. Tasks were not siloed. Nurses and techs alike answered call bells, responded to alarms, and supported each other. It was not about hierarchy — it was about shared responsibility.

3. Open Communication

There was a steady, respectful exchange of information between nurses and techs. Issues were identified early, addressed openly, and met with quick, coordinated plans.

The result was better care, smoother workflow, and greater peace of mind.

Compared to her previous unit, this one felt intentional, inclusive, and truly patient-centered. It was a welcome change — one that reminded Theresa why she became a nurse in the first place.

At the end of her shift, she jokingly asked the Charge Nurse if the unit was hiring. The response she received surprised her. The process was unlike anything she had encountered on her current unit.

"Yes, we're hiring," the Charge Nurse said. "But it's a process. First, you shadow on the unit to get a feel for how we work. Then you'll interview with one of our managers, followed by a group interview with nurses, a patient care technician, and one of the unit secretaries. We want to make sure every new hire is a good fit. After that, our unit educator assesses your learning style so we can match you with a preceptor who helps you grow. And during orientation, you're required to attend at least one Unit Council meeting to see how we solve problems as a team."

As Theresa returned to her home unit to grab her belongings from her locker, she shook her head in disbelief. The contrast was jarring. Six call lights were blinking. Two phones rang nonstop. A bed alarm blared down the hall. Yet four team members sat idly, unmoved by the chaos around them.

That night, Theresa opened her laptop and began updating her resume. She wasn't just ready for a new job. She was ready for a new culture — one where she didn't merely survive the shift but felt proud to be part of something better.

People don't usually quit jobs. They quit cultures.

Between 2020 and 2024, an average of 25.9% of bedside nurses either left their current unit, transferred elsewhere, or exited the healthcare facility entirely. For new graduates, the number was nearly 18% within their first year of practice (ANA, 2023).

We've read the definition of culture in textbooks, journals, and continuing education modules. It's been stated time and time again, culture is the collection of attitudes, beliefs, and behaviors that shape the everyday atmosphere of a workplace. And while it may feel intangible, here's the truth:

Every single person on your unit shapes the culture.

That includes you — the person holding this book right now.

You have the power to influence your unit's culture for the better.

"Isn't that the Nurse Manager's job?"

In some ways, yes. Nurse Managers, whether they realize it or not, are constantly shaping experiences that influence culture — through who they promote, how they implement policies, how they lead meetings, and how they respond to feedback.

Those experiences build beliefs.

And those beliefs drive behavior.

(Connors & Smith, 2011)

Managers hold influence. They provide resources, set expectations, and carry enormous responsibility.

But they are not the culture.

The culture is made up of the people working side by side, shift after shift.

It's your beliefs.

It's your experiences.

It's your interactions with one another.

That's where culture lives.

And that's where it can change.

GUIDELINES FOR SHIFTING CULTURE

1. Accountability

Let's clear something up: accountability isn't punishment. It's empowerment through ownership. It means knowing you have a responsibility to your patients, your teammates, and yourself. Nurses practice this every single day — whether it's catching a colleague's mistake and addressing it, covering for someone who's tied up in a room, or working together to keep patients safe. Most hospitals even have reporting systems like Quantros or Safe Connect, where you can document concerns — yours or a teammate's — without fear of retaliation.

Why? Because the safest care comes from people who take ownership of their mindset and actions. These are the nurses who double-check, speak up early, and never assume someone else will handle it.

When you lead by example, others take notice. And many will follow.

Actionable Ways to Practice Accountability

a. Meet Expectations

Your Nurse Manager sets the expectations. It's your responsibility to meet them.

How often do we hear the same reminders in huddles? Prevent falls. Keep up with pain reassessments. Be thorough in your charting.

They might sound repetitive, but these aren't just rules. They're safeguards for your patients and sanity-savers for your team.

- *Reframe your mindset:* Instead of rolling your eyes, ask, "What can I control right now?"
- *Stay present:* Don't just check tasks off a list. Own the outcomes.
- *Be proactive:* Before leaving a high-fall-risk patient's room, check the bed alarm, put down floor pads, and make sure the call light is within reach. Those extra seconds can prevent a serious incident.

That kind of ownership builds trust. And it saves lives.

b. Open Communication

A healthy team communicates – honestly, clearly, and respectfully.

Closed communication (hoarding information, vague updates, avoiding conflict) creates confusion, tension, and mistrust. Open and consistent dialogue builds trust, reduces friction, and makes difficult shifts a little easier to get through.

Start small. Be curious. Listen fully before responding. That one habit can shift the energy on your entire unit.

And remember – patients count on transparency too. When you're giving meds, updating them on their plan of care, or explaining a procedure, they rely on you to be clear and honest. That same openness should carry over to how we speak to each other at work.

The Three Pillars of Open Communication

There's no magic checklist, but these three principles are your foundation:

a. Trust

Nothing works without it. Trust begins with active listening – being present when someone speaks. That means making eye contact, paraphrasing what you heard, and checking to make sure you understood.

Example:

"So you're saying the med wasn't documented, but it was given? Got it. Let's fix that now."

That small exchange builds clarity and trust.

b. Context

Context turns a comment into a conversation. Move past yes-or-no questions and dig a little deeper.

- "How did that make you feel?"
- "Can you walk me through what happened?"
- "Help me understand your take on it."

These open-ended questions show that you care and help create space for real conversation — especially when tension is high.

c. Congruence

Good communication isn't a one-time effort. It's a daily habit. The calm, supportive tone you use with patients? Bring that same energy to your coworkers. Consistency builds respect. Over time, it changes culture.

Giving Feedback: The Culture-Builder

Toxic work environments thrive in silence.

When bad habits or negative attitudes go unchecked, stress builds. Frustration festers. Mistrust grows. And eventually, people leave.

But it doesn't have to get that far.

1. Make It Timely

Don't let issues linger. Address them while they're still fresh. Avoiding conflict only makes things worse. A calm check-in today can prevent a blowup tomorrow.

2. Be Clear and Direct

Pick the right time — during a handoff, in a quiet hallway, or after a shift — and be concise. Focus on the behavior and how it affects the team or patient care. Stick to facts. Clarity is your best tool.

3. Use Real Examples

Avoid exaggerations like "always" or "never." They put people on the defensive. Instead, share specific, recent examples.

Example:

"Yesterday and today, I noticed you didn't answer call lights for Room 412. It left the rest of us scrambling. Can we talk about what's going on?"

That's direct, respectful, and fair.

4. Stay Cool

Giving feedback is not a license to vent. Stay focused. Keep it professional. Don't bring up old history. If emotions run high — yours or theirs — pause, breathe, and refocus. A calm approach is how things actually get better.

Accepting Feedback

In *Thanks for the Feedback*, Douglas Stone and Sheila Heen explore how to become a better receiver of feedback so you can integrate it more effectively into both your work and personal life. Strengthening this skill not only improves your performance but also fosters healthier, more trusting relationships with those around you.

The biggest challenge in receiving feedback is managing the emotional response it can trigger. Strong reactions can cloud your judgment and make it difficult to truly hear and process what's being said. By recognizing what tends to set you off – and understanding how your emotional wiring influences your response – you can begin to manage those reactions with more clarity and intention.

Common Feedback Triggers

Truth Trigger

When this trigger is activated, we reject the content of the feedback, labeling it as wrong, unfair, or irrelevant. The antidote is to pause before reacting. Use that brief moment to reflect objectively and consider whether there may be some truth underneath the discomfort.

Relationship Trigger

This occurs when we focus more on who is giving the feedback than on what is being said. Instead of evaluating the message, we let our feelings about the person cloud our judgment. Moving past this trigger means separating the message from the messenger. Focus on the content, not the relationship dynamic. (*Stone & Heen, 2015*)

A Three-Step Method for Approaching Feedback

1. Accept It

Practice active listening. Stay present, open, and engaged. Assume the person's intent is to solve a problem or offer support, not to criticize or attack.

2. Analyze It

Ask clarifying questions. Request specific examples to better understand the feedback. Reflect honestly: Have I shown this behavior before? Could this be something I need to work on?

3. Act on It

Depending on your relationship with the feedback giver, ask for suggestions on next steps. If needed, consult with a mentor, supervisor, or trusted peer. Then, decide how you will apply what you've learned.

Progressively Role Modeling Behavior

You don't need to master these communication skills overnight. As your nursing career progresses, you'll have many opportunities to practice and refine them in daily interactions. Every small effort helps shift the culture of your unit toward one rooted in accountability, collaboration, and mutual respect.

When you address issues directly, own your mistakes, and follow through on solutions, you uplift the entire team. This kind of leadership doesn't require a title or recognition. It quietly builds trust, earns long-term respect, and leaves a lasting impact on those around you.

Conflict Resolution

Even with the best intentions, conflict is inevitable. Sometimes it escalates to the point where management or Human Resources must intervene. In nursing, conflict typically appears in three forms: peer-to-peer disputes, cliques, and toxic leadership dynamics.

Common Behaviors in Difficult Team Members

Here are some recognizable behaviors displayed by challenging colleagues:

1. Constant negativity, such as frequent complaining or criticism
2. Gossip and rumor-spreading that damage trust and morale
3. Passive-aggressive remarks or backhanded compliments
4. Bullying or intimidation tactics
5. Emotional volatility, including mood swings or outbursts
6. Lack of collaboration or unwillingness to assist the team

Just as every team brings a variety of strengths, it also includes a range of personalities. Some colleagues lift others up, while others create tension or conflict. Recognizing the patterns in problematic behavior allows you to respond with more intention, set healthy boundaries, and communicate more effectively.

Ultimately, every interaction is a chance to create a workplace where people can contribute meaningfully, grow professionally, and feel supported.

Navigating Difficult Peer-to-Peer Conflicts: Actionable Steps

These steps will help you build and apply the interpersonal skills needed to manage tough workplace relationships.

1. Don't Avoid Crucial Conversations

Many people fear that addressing problematic behavior will escalate the issue. In reality, avoiding it almost always makes things worse. Unspoken frustrations build up and begin to affect how you see the other person. That quiet resentment seeps into your tone, attitude, and even body language. Eventually, the tension impacts not just your relationship but the entire team.

As Grenny et al. (2021) emphasize, the longer you delay difficult conversations, the more damage is done. Often, the best path forward is also the most uncomfortable one: start the conversation early.

A one-on-one talk may feel awkward, but it can help realign expectations and clear the air. The discomfort is temporary. The potential for a stronger, more respectful working relationship makes it worth it.

2. Set Clear Boundaries

Boundaries are not selfish. They are essential. They protect your peace, preserve your energy, and foster professional respect.

Start by changing your mindset. You are not being difficult by setting boundaries; you are being clear about how you expect to be treated. Communicate them with confidence and consistency. Without boundaries, burnout and resentment grow. With boundaries, you create a healthier foundation for respectful connections.

People treat you based on what you allow. Boundaries are how you teach others what is acceptable.

3. Seek Help When Necessary

If a private conversation feels overwhelming, ask your manager to arrange a facilitated meeting. Having a neutral third party helps ensure the discussion stays respectful and focused on resolution.

If you are unsure how to hold boundaries or initiate a conversation, seek advice from someone you respect—a veteran nurse, mentor, or preceptor. They can offer practical insights for approaching the situation professionally.

Addressing Cliques in the Workplace

Cliques are tight-knit social circles that often exclude others. At first, these friendships may seem harmless. But left unchecked, they can create toxic dynamics where favoritism thrives, morale suffers, and divisions form.

According to a CareerBuilder study, nearly 45 percent of employees report the presence of cliques at work (McGovern, 2023).

Their main weapon is exclusion—and it can sting. These groups may monopolize prime assignments, dominate social spaces, or intentionally isolate others. In healthcare, this behavior does more than hurt feelings. It can put patient safety at risk.

At their worst, cliques cover for each other's mistakes, withhold help from teammates, and even engage in unethical or unsafe practices. When management tolerates this, the outcome is predictable: high turnover, broken trust, and a fractured team.

Eventually, the impact of clique behavior becomes visible to everyone—not just those directly affected.

Actionable Steps to Address Cliques

- **Address It Directly**

  Speak up. You do not have to be confrontational—just clear and factual. Explain why certain behaviors are harmful and how they affect team culture.

- **Expect Pushback**

  Clique members often overreact when challenged. If they get defensive or dramatic, remind yourself that their reaction reflects them, not you. Stay calm and composed. Do not escalate.

- **Be Specific**

  Use recent, concrete examples. Mention the date, action, and impact. Reinforce the shared goal of patient care and express your expectation for fairness and collaboration.

Standing up to clique behavior weakens its power. It also shows others that toxic dynamics can and should be confronted.

If the issue involves someone in a leadership role, you may need to take a more formal route. We will explore that next.

Navigating Toxic Leadership

Toxic leadership involves repeated patterns of abusive, manipulative, or harmful behavior by those in positions of authority. This undermines employee well-being and can derail an entire unit. Toxic leaders often focus on their own power or image rather than team success, using fear, intimidation, or favoritism to stay in control.

These leaders may show narcissistic traits—exaggerated self-importance and a lack of empathy. They reject feedback, take criticism personally, and dismiss new ideas as threats. Over time, they build a culture of fear where staff feel afraid to speak up or suggest improvements (Ofei et al., 2023).

Modern leadership theory outlines four core management styles, first introduced by German psychologist Kurt Lewin (1939) and later expanded by Bernard Bass (1990). These styles help us understand effective leadership—and identify when it turns toxic.

Common Leadership Styles in Healthcare

1. Autocratic

   The manager makes all decisions independently. This top-down approach, also called micromanaging, often suppresses initiative and trust.

2. Democratic

   The manager encourages input and fosters collaboration. This inclusive style builds morale, supports problem-solving, and gives team members a voice.

3. Laissez-faire

   A hands-off approach that allows significant autonomy. It works well with highly skilled, self-motivated teams that do not need constant oversight.

4. Transformational

    This leader sets high standards, models dedication, and inspires growth. Transformational leaders empower their teams and hold themselves accountable along with others.

In practice, most managers blend these styles depending on the situation. However, toxic nurse managers tend to do the opposite of what effective leadership requires. Their behavior may involve one or more of the following harmful traits:

Characteristics of Toxic Leadership

Micromanagement – Excessive control, refusal to delegate, and a lack of trust in the team's abilities often define this trait.

Verbal Abuse and Intimidation – Yelling, bullying, issuing threats, or speaking in a condescending tone—whether in person or through hostile emails—signals a clear lack of respect.

Low Emotional Intelligence – According to Daniel Goleman (1998), emotional intelligence includes self-awareness, self-management, social awareness, and relationship management. Toxic leaders often lack these qualities. They make impulsive decisions, ignore the emotional impact of their actions, or mishandle interpersonal conflict.

Narcissism and Lack of Accountability – These managers may be more concerned with personal image than with team well-being. They often ignore the organization's mission, deflect responsibility, and blame others for mistakes. They may take credit for team successes using "I," while ignoring the contributions of others (Kimura, 2003). Some go further by creating inner circles of like-minded staff who reinforce their behavior.

If you are dealing with a toxic work dynamic, know this: simply tolerating it is not the answer. Long-term exposure to a hostile environment can lead to burnout, anxiety, depression, reduced productivity, and higher turnover.

Here is the good news—you are not powerless. There are practical steps you can take to protect yourself and create change.

Actionable Steps for Addressing Toxic Leadership

1. Clarify Intent with Contrasting

When approaching difficult conversations, use a communication strategy called *Contrasting*. This method helps reduce misunderstandings by pairing a "Don't/Do" format:

- The "Don't" part anticipates the other person's fear or concern.
- The "Do" part clarifies your true intent and reinforces respect.

(Grenny et al., 2021)

Example 1

"I don't want you to take this the wrong way, but during today's huddle, this was the third time this week you pointed out a documentation error I made. I've noticed similar errors from others that weren't mentioned. I do want feedback, but I'm concerned about how it's being delivered."

Example 2

"Last week, you brushed off a concern I raised about feedback passed to me secondhand. I don't think that helps our working relationship. I do want to address any issues directly, just not through the grapevine."

Using a contrasting statement helps clarify that you are seeking resolution, not conflict. While some behavior may appear toxic, it could also stem from stress or miscommunication. Choosing a calm, private moment to talk increases the chances of a productive outcome.

If the situation continues or crosses the line into abusive conduct, it is appropriate to say so and to explain the effect it has on your ability to work—or your emotional well-being outside of work.

Speak to the behavior, not the person. Offer specific, recent examples. If needed, include a neutral witness. Some organizations require attempts at direct resolution before escalating to Human Resources.

2. Review Workplace Policies

If direct communication feels unsafe or does not lead to change, review your organization's policies on harassment and conduct. Reach out to Human Resources for clarification. They can provide written definitions and guide you through the proper procedures.

Ask questions such as:

- What qualifies as a reportable offense?
- Are there steps that must be taken before escalating the issue?
- What protections exist for staff who report misconduct?

Some organizations start with informal discussions or verbal warnings and escalate based on the situation. Policies vary, so understanding yours is key.

3. Document, Document, Document

If the issue persists, begin keeping a private record of events. Your documentation should include:

- Date and time
- Description of the behavior
- Names of witnesses, if any
- Quotes or emails (use screenshots if needed)

This log will be critical if formal action becomes necessary. Knowing how your workplace defines misconduct will help ensure your documentation is relevant and effective.

Remember, reporting toxic leadership may mean confronting those who hired or enabled that leader. Expect resistance—but stay firm. You have the right to protect your work environment and mental health.

4. Use the Chain of Command

If the issue continues to escalate, reach out to your manager's supervisor—often the Associate Director or

Director of Nursing—and notify HR as well. Be clear and professional. Explain your concerns and share the steps you've already taken to resolve the issue.

5. Rally Support from Colleagues

If leadership remains unresponsive, speak with trusted team members. Chances are, others are having similar experiences. When multiple voices come together, the message becomes harder to ignore.

Collective action increases visibility and can create the momentum needed to bring about meaningful change.

Job Satisfaction: A Powerful Buffer

When nurses feel supported and valued, they tend to be more engaged, less prone to burnout, and more likely to stay in their roles. In fact, job satisfaction can act as a protective barrier against the harmful effects of toxic leadership (Ofei et al., 2023).

Tools That Can Transform Culture

- Accountability
- Constructive Feedback
- Conflict Resolution
- Self-Advocacy

These are not just corporate buzzwords. They are essential tools for building a healthy and productive work environment.

You should never feel pressured to leave a job you love because of one person's poor behavior. While walking away might feel like the easiest option, these tools give you the power to create change from within.

Toxic leadership is not limited to certain services or specialties. It is a widespread challenge across the healthcare system. But with resilience, strong communication, and a clear sense of boundaries, you can protect both your career and your colleagues.

Given the ongoing national nursing shortage, retaining skilled and committed nurses has never been more critical.

Your voice, your well-being, and your experience matter.

N2

COUNCILS

A single leaf working alone provides no shade."
— Chuck Page

N2 COUNCILS

Unit-Based Councils (UBCs) are among the most underutilized yet powerful self-directed tools nurses can leverage to reduce turnover and improve working conditions. The concept of shared governance in nursing was brought into the spotlight in 1985 with the publication of *Shared Governance for Nursing: A Creative Approach to Professional Accountability*. Authors Tim Porter-O'Grady and Sharon Finnigan defined shared governance as "a structural model through which nurses can express and manage their practice with a higher level of professional autonomy."

In practical terms, shared governance creates a collaborative partnership between nursing staff, leadership, interdisciplinary colleagues, and other healthcare team members. Its aim is to foster open communication, shared decision-making, professional accountability, and a culture of nursing excellence. A Unit-Based Council empowers nurses to take ownership of their environment, propose and implement improvements, and contribute meaningfully to both team culture and patient care. Crucially, shared governance is not intended to burden nurses with additional tasks. Instead, it offers a structure that helps deliver patient-centered care while making the work environment better for everyone involved.

When used effectively, UBCs can elevate job satisfaction, promote professional development, and strengthen collaboration among staff within healthcare teams.

How Unit-Based Councils Fit into Shared Governance

UBCs form the backbone of shared governance structures in many hospitals. These councils are typically composed of interdisciplinary team members representing specific units or combination of units making up a service. Their primary role is to offer a consistent, structured platform where staff can express concerns, collaborate on solutions, identify areas for growth, and contribute directly to decisions that shape their work environment and impact patient care (CHCM, 2023).

The role of the UBC often scales based on a facility's size and available clinical and educational support. In larger institutions, UBCs are frequently integrated into broader networks of professional practice councils.

At a 437-bed medical facility, for instance, UBCs function as part of six other professional practice councils. This model enables nurses to collaborate across units and engage with peers throughout the organization.

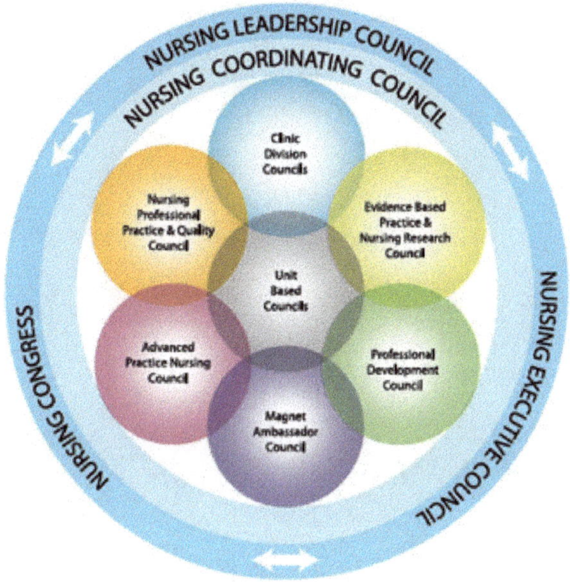

At a smaller 139-bed hospital, each of the seven nursing units maintains its own UBC. The chairpersons of these councils meet as part of a Professional Nursing Practice Council (PNPC), where they exchange feedback and ideas on clinical standards, quality improvement initiatives, staff development goals, and nursing research efforts.

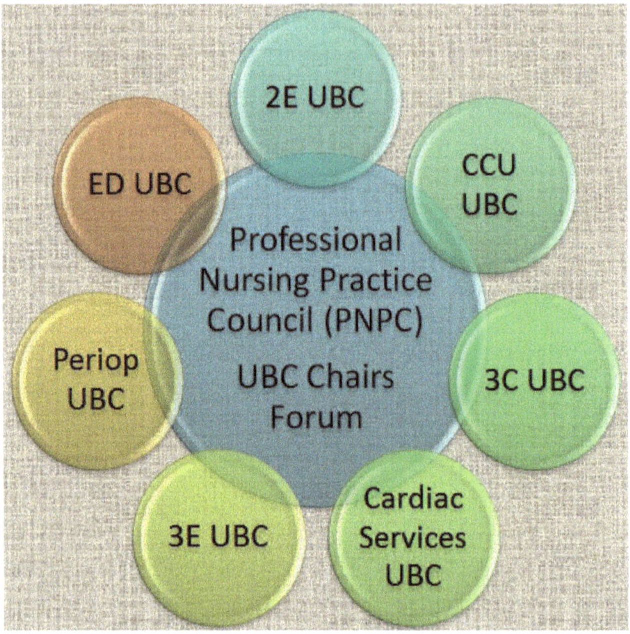

Guidelines for Creating and Strengthening a Unit-Based Council

The following steps are designed to help you form, improve, or manage a Unit-Based Council (UBC). These are not rigid rules but adaptable guidelines that can be tailored to meet your unit's needs while aligning with your facility's shared governance structure.

For units without an active UBC:

- Form a small exploratory committee to determine the council's intended role.
- Review current decision-making and communication methods on your unit.
- Discuss which policies, processes, or challenges the UBC should prioritize.

It is also important to plan for leadership continuity to ensure council roles transition smoothly. (For more, see the Continuity Framework in Chapter Six)

Once these discussions are complete, the committee should:

1. Create a mission statement that reflects your unit's shared governance goals.
2. Draft bylaws outlining the UBC's structure and purpose.
3. Propose a revised nursing leadership framework that incorporates UBC positions.
4. Establish a reliable method for communicating council updates and decisions to all staff.
5. Appoint an advisor for the council, typically a Nurse Manager, Associate Director or comparable leadership position.
6. Announce open positions and hold elections for Chairperson and Co-Chairperson.
7. Host the first official meeting, using a Goals and Solutions Framework to begin addressing key challenges.

Actionable Steps for Building a Successful UBC

When creating or restructuring a UBC, it's essential to energize your team around its purpose and communicate the benefits of participation. Emphasize how the council supports nurses personally and professionally, from influencing policy to improving work satisfaction.

Encourage staff to nominate themselves or peers for UBC roles. Leaders may need to actively promote the long-term value of nurse-led change. A strong council takes time and commitment. Leadership may initiate the effort, but sustained success depends on motivated team members willing to serve as catalysts for improvement.

In healthcare, effective change agents often share key traits — optimism, resilience, empathy, and a collaborative mindset — that help foster lasting success (Berta & Ciriani, 2022).

Recommended UBC Structure and Roles

Chairperson

An elected nurse who presides over meetings, partners with unit leadership, and acts as a liaison to other UBCs and professional councils. This role involves leading discussions, overseeing projects, and maintaining open communication with staff.

Co-Chairperson

Also elected, the Co-Chair supports the Chairperson, records meeting minutes, co-manages projects, and facilitates interdisciplinary coordination. For example, they might collaborate with a respiratory therapist to address training needs for ventilator care.

Day and Night Shift Facilitators

These nurses represent staff feedback from their respective shifts and bring issues to the council and leadership. Topics may include workflow improvements or professionalism. Facilitators are also responsible for sharing updates with their teams.

Advisor

Typically the Nurse Manager, Associate Director of Nursing, or another leader. Advisors join the end of meetings to allow members time for open discussion before providing guidance, resources, or feedback on council goals.

UBC Members

Any staff member interested in improving the unit and driving positive change.

Elections and Nominations

Chairperson and Co-Chairperson roles can be nominated by any unit member, including self-nominations. Elections should be supervised by the Nurse Manager. Facilitators are nominated by staff from their shift and voted in during a shift-specific election, also overseen by the Nurse Manager.

Laws That Govern

Once leadership roles are filled, bylaws should be created to define how the council will operate. These should include:

1. Clearly defined leadership responsibilities.
2. A meeting schedule and rules for conducting meetings.
3. Term limits and procedures for replacing members who step down.

4. Guidelines for addressing submitted issues, with transparent communication to encourage staff participation and clarify timelines.
5. A voting process for policy changes, including the required number of votes to pass proposals.

Obtaining Information for Change

Communication is key. UBCs are a vital platform for staff to voice concerns and offer ideas. To be effective, councils must provide clear and accessible ways for staff to submit issues or feedback.

Hospitals can use suggestion boxes, digital platforms, or forums to collect and track concerns. Standardizing submissions improves clarity and helps the council prioritize.

Effective communication methods include:

- Pre-shift huddles
- Informal one-on-one conversations
- Anonymous suggestion forms on shared digital platforms
- Unit-based surveys, either broad or topic-specific

Surveys are a practical tool for understanding staff needs and perspectives. They can be shared through email, QR codes posted in common areas, or links on the unit's internal site. Anonymity encourages honest input from staff who may feel hesitant to speak up.

Once feedback is collected, the Chairperson should review the data and identify the top actionable items.

Issues that appear repeatedly – especially those affecting patient care, training, or standardized procedures – should be prioritized for the next meeting's agenda.

Staying on Task and Offering Flexible Attendance Options

Council meetings are led by the Chairperson. In some units, a dedicated secretary records meeting minutes, while in others, this task falls to the Co-Chair or a designated member. In most meetings, the Advisor joins only for the final five to ten minutes. This structure encourages open discussion among members, including honest conversations about leadership concerns.

Although meeting times and dates are typically outlined in the council bylaws, they should remain flexible to accommodate the needs of staff. Members should have the option to attend in person or virtually, using secure smartphone apps or teleconferencing tools. Offering compensation for meeting attendance, when possible, can also boost participation.

To maximize attendance, schedule meetings around shift transitions, such as at 07:30 or 08:00. This timing allows both night and day shift nurses to join after giving patient reports. The Charge Nurse, Nurse Educator, or other staff can help ensure the unit remains covered during these times.

Meetings should be positive, focused, and efficient. The Chairperson is responsible for minimizing distractions and keeping the group on task. Each meeting should follow a clear agenda with a structured order and time limits for each topic. The Chair and Co-Chair work together to maintain focus and address any off-topic or disruptive behavior as needed.

To improve efficiency, facilitators should submit updates in advance so the Chair can present them clearly. After committee updates, the council moves into discussion of unit-specific issues. The Advisor then joins the meeting to review decisions made and provide feedback or guidance on next steps.

Emphasizing Accountability, Engagement, and Multidisciplinary Involvement

Leaders play a key role in fostering team engagement. By actively inviting staff to contribute ideas and participate in decision-making, they help build a culture of trust, psychological safety, and collaboration. The more involved staff feel, the more likely they are to stay committed and invested in the unit's success.

It is equally important to follow through on feedback. Listening without action sends the message that input is not valued. Even if a suggestion is controversial or lacks full agreement, it should be addressed respectfully. When team members see that their voices influence outcomes, it fosters ownership and accountability.

Author's Note:

A common challenge I've observed in these settings is what I call the *Group Emulator Effect*. This happens when individuals, uncertain of their standing within the group, repeat familiar ideas simply to avoid judgment or exclusion. It is often a sign that psychological safety is lacking.

Staff must feel confident expressing authentic opinions. This is not easy. Speaking up against the group can lead to being labeled difficult or rebellious. Yet, in my experience, these dissenting voices are often the ones that drive real change and help root out toxic behaviors that may otherwise go unchecked.

The Importance of Multidisciplinary Team Involvement

A multidisciplinary team member is any healthcare professional from a different discipline who contributes to patient care. This includes Respiratory Therapists, Social Workers, Physician Assistants, Nurse Practitioners, and others. Their perspectives often help resolve complex unit challenges by providing specialized knowledge or suggesting new approaches.

When a particular issue arises, inviting the relevant professional to attend a UBC meeting can be highly beneficial. These contributors may not only help solve problems but also serve as ongoing educational resources for the team.

Even non-clinical staff—such as dietary services, environmental services, or bed management—can play a vital role in the unit's performance. Their work, although not always directly tied to patient care, can significantly affect patient experience and unit flow. Including them in relevant discussions enhances cooperation and strengthens the team.

Fostering multidisciplinary collaboration promotes mutual respect, deepens understanding between roles, and aligns the unit around the shared goal of high-quality, patient-centered care.

Project Roadmaps

Project roadmaps give UBCs a clear and structured way to address problems on the unit. These visual planning tools help teams stay organized as they work through each stage of a project. A well-developed roadmap outlines goals, timelines, responsibilities, and benchmarks for success.

By using roadmaps, councils can ensure accountability, maintain momentum, and track meaningful progress. These tools help teams stay focused, adapt when needed, and achieve tangible outcomes that benefit both staff and patients.

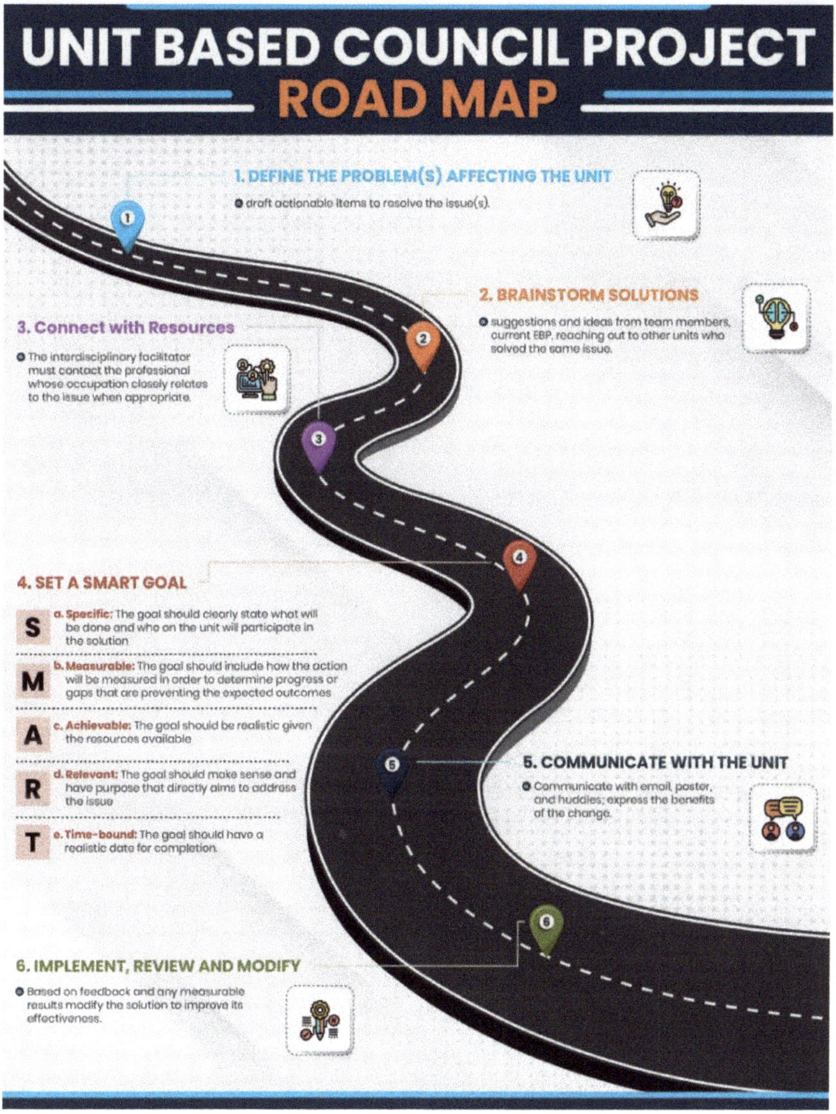

1. Define the Problem(s) Affecting the Unit

a. Using the data collected on unit-related issues, draft the top three actionable items that require resolution. Prioritize them based on their impact on patient care, staff workflow, and safety.

2. Brainstorm Solutions

a. Gather suggestions and feedback from team members. Consider incorporating evidence-based practices from clinical journals, textbooks, or by consulting with other units that have addressed similar challenges.

b. Utilize the expertise of the Unit Educator and Nurse Manager to expand possible solutions.

3. Connect with Resources

a. The interdisciplinary facilitator (Co-Chair) should reach out to professionals whose expertise directly relates to the issue at hand.

b. Depending on the shared governance model in place, involve other councils—such as Development-Based or Evidence-Based Practice Councils—to help eliminate barriers and refine interventions.

4. Set a SMART Goal

- Specific: Clearly define what will be done and who is responsible.
- Measurable: Identify how progress and results will be tracked.
- Achievable: Ensure the goal is realistic given the resources available.
- Relevant: The goal must directly address the identified issue and align with the unit's priorities.
- Time-bound: Establish a firm and realistic timeline for completion.

5. Communicate with the Unit

Announce the solution plan and timeline. Use multiple communication channels—such as emails, posters, huddles, and staff meetings—to ensure all staff understand the importance of the intervention and the anticipated benefits.

6. Implement, Review, and Modify

- After implementation, collect staff feedback and evaluate outcomes using the predetermined metrics.
- Modify the plan as necessary to enhance effectiveness.
- Continue updating the unit on progress, milestones, and outcomes to maintain engagement and support.

Solutions in Action:

A busy 26-bed Medical-Surgical Unit was struggling with inconsistency in bedside reporting. The lack of a shared understanding led to fragmented practices:

- Some nurses gave report at the nurse's station.
- Others reported from the doorway without patient involvement.

This inconsistency created several recurring issues:

1. Patient Care Gaps: Patients were often found soiled shortly after shift change, disrupting early-shift responsibilities.
2. IV Pump Errors: Medication pumps were either misprogrammed, had a small amount of fluid left in

the bag adding an additional task for the oncoming nurse to complete or in some cases turned off.

3. Fall Risks: Bed alarms were left inactive, contributing to actual falls and near misses.

With ongoing staff dissatisfaction and reliance on float nurses unfamiliar with expectations, the unit re-established its Unit-Based Council to address the problem directly. The council developed a standardized bedside report protocol, leading to a series of strategic changes:

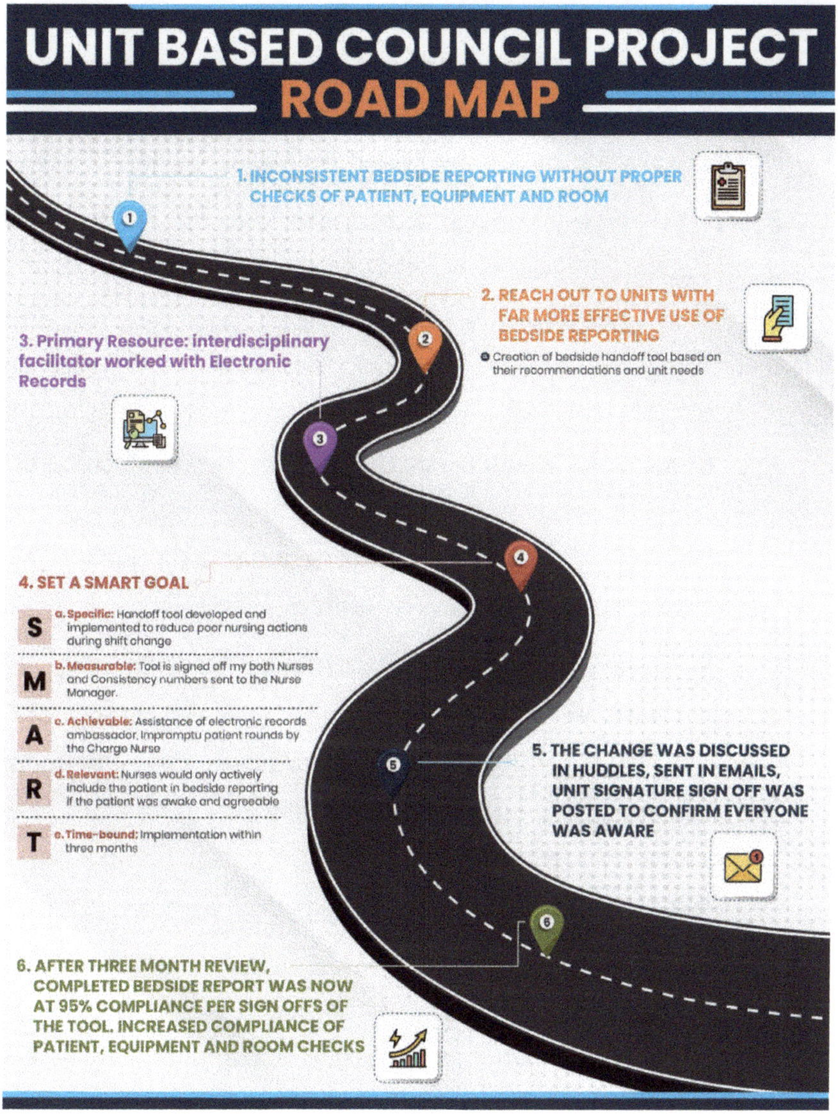

1. The Unit-Based Council (UBC) established clear, agreed-upon steps for completing bedside reporting in line with hospital policy. These steps were tailored to meet the needs of the unit's patient population and were informed by feedback from

two unit-wide surveys and several pre-shift huddle discussions. Once finalized and approved through a vote, the steps were announced via posters, emails, and a scheduled implementation date.

2. The team consulted other units that had demonstrated strong bedside reporting practices. One particularly effective suggestion was to integrate a bedside handoff tool into the electronic health record system. Created by the facility's Electronic Record Ambassador, this tool allowed both nurses to confirm task completion by signing off digitally. Nurse Managers could then access this data to monitor compliance.
3. A new protocol was introduced to only include patients in bedside reports if they were awake and receptive. Patients had expressed fatigue from repeated reports throughout the day. When patients were asleep, nurses focused on safety checks while avoiding unnecessary disruptions to rest.
4. For patients unable to reposition themselves, both the outgoing and incoming nurses worked together to reposition the patient and assess for incontinence during the safety check.
5. Continuous intravenous medications were verified for accuracy against provider orders. If a bag was within ten percent of completion, the outgoing nurse replaced it before ending their shift.

6. Bed alarms and related safety devices were checked by the oncoming nurse. Both nurses confirmed that alarms for chairs or lap belts were set appropriately for use during the next shift.
7. The Charge Nurse conducted random patient rounds to verify that bedside reports were completed and to gather patient feedback. Any staff who refused to participate in bedside reporting were reported to leadership.
8. This structured process proved so effective that it was adopted by other units with similar patient populations.
9. Within a short period, bedside report compliance rose to 95 percent based on electronic sign-offs. Overnight-to-morning fall rates dropped significantly, medication errors were sharply reduced, and overall morale and unit cohesion greatly improved.

Solutions in Action:

An eighteen-bed acute care pulmonary unit faced a range of performance issues, primarily due to over half the nursing staff having less than two years of experience. Many team members were unfamiliar with the specific needs of Otolaryngology (Ear, Nose, and Throat) patients, as well as the specialized equipment and bedside procedures involved.

1. This lack of familiarity led to frequent frustration among the surgical team, who found patient care orders either incomplete or incorrectly executed.

2. Respiratory Therapists also expressed concern over a high volume of non-urgent pages and calls. Many of these involved basic equipment troubleshooting that should have been handled by nursing staff.
3. The varying experience levels on the team created additional tension. Less experienced nurses believed that higher-acuity patients should be assigned to the more experienced staff. This resulted in passive-aggressive behavior, gossip, and reduced teamwork. Absenteeism also increased as stress levels rose.

In response, the newly hired Nurse Manager organized a series of cluster meetings, grouping nurses by experience level—high, moderate, and new. Each group was invited to identify their most pressing challenges. The Unit-Based Council was then encouraged to take the lead in generating actionable solutions, with the manager offering resources and guidance to support their efforts.

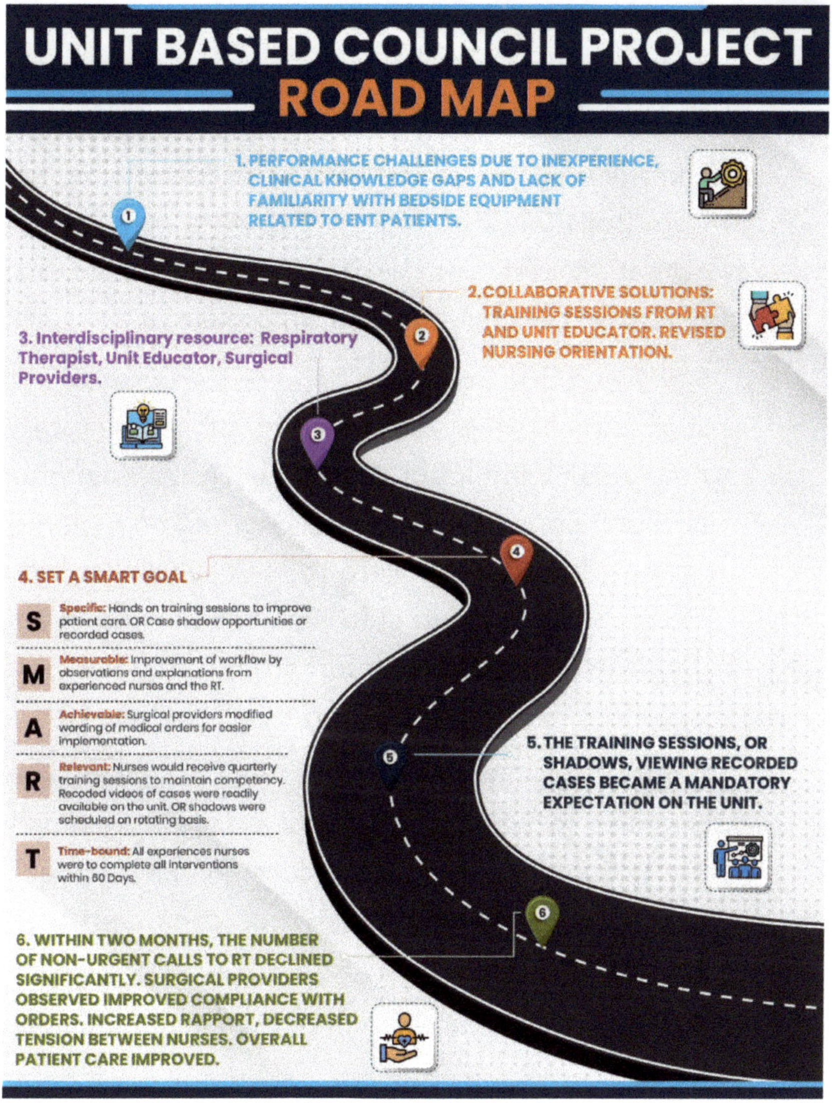

The UBC initiated the process by:

The Unit-Based Council (UBC) took several targeted steps to address the performance issues on the pulmonary unit:

1. Inviting Key Stakeholders: Surgical providers and Respiratory Therapists were invited to a

collaborative meeting where they shared concerns and offered recommendations for practical, mutually supported solutions.

2. Engaging Experienced Staff: Seasoned nurses from both day and night shifts were consulted to gather insight into workflow inefficiencies and opportunities for process improvement.
3. Reviewing and Voting on Solutions: Feedback and suggestions were discussed in subsequent UBC meetings. With input from the Nurse Manager and Unit Educator, the council agreed on a plan of action. The solutions were formally voted on, then clearly communicated to the full nursing team. The Nurse Manager reinforced that the new care approach would be adopted by all staff members.
4. Introducing Targeted Education: Nurses were required to watch procedural videos to reinforce understanding of bedside care for ENT patients and build foundational clinical competence.
5. Providing Hands-On Training: Respiratory Therapists partnered with the Unit Educator to lead training sessions on various types of equipment, troubleshooting methods, patient care techniques, and proper order management. During these sessions, the Nurse Educator identified inconsistencies in the orientation process that were contributing to knowledge gaps. Orientation

procedures were revised to deliver clearer and more consistent onboarding information for new hires.

6. Clarifying Medical Orders: Surgical providers attended a UBC meeting where they worked alongside nursing staff to adjust the wording of several medical orders. The revised language made instructions easier to understand and execute accurately across the team.

Measurable Outcomes

Within just three months of rolling out these interventions:

- Non-urgent calls to Respiratory Therapy decreased significantly.
- The surgical team noted substantial improvements in the quality and consistency of patient care.
- Tensions among nurses over patient assignments and acuity levels diminished.
- The UBC sustained momentum by developing new project roadmaps focused on performance enhancement and interdisciplinary collaboration.

In Summary

Unit-Based Shared Governance Council (UBC) initiatives empower healthcare professionals to take ownership of their practice, enhance job satisfaction, and uphold excellence in patient-centered care. By integrating shared governance principles, hospitals cultivate a culture of collaboration, elevate clinical outcomes, and give voice to staff at every level — from leadership to frontline caregivers.

Through thoughtful planning and active engagement, UBCs can spark lasting improvements that reinforce high standards across the healthcare system (CHCM, 2023).

N3
COACHING (PRECEPTING)

"Coaching is about enabling individuals to make conscious decisions and empowering them to become leaders in their own lives."
- Dr. Maria Nemeth

03

N3
COACHING (PRECEPTING)

As Natalie sat in her Nurse Manager's office, resignation letter in hand, she was struck by how different this moment felt compared to the day of her interview. Back then, after a four-hour shadow shift, she had been filled with excitement. Now, just five months into her first nursing job, she was quitting. And it hurt more than she expected.

"So, what do you think was the biggest factor in your decision?" her manager asked gently.

"The six different preceptors," Natalie replied without hesitation. "My confidence is gone. I feel completely lost when I'm on the unit. Every one of them had their own style, their own expectations. And with each new person, I felt like I was starting over. Some were downright unfriendly. Even rude."

"I understand your frustrations, Natalie," her manager began. "But we've been short-staffed. Your first preceptor went on maternity leave, which we had discussed. Then your second had to take time off for personal reasons."

"I get that," Natalie interrupted, "but the ones I've had since then weren't a good fit either. One had less than a year of experience herself. She made a med error, and I noticed it, but I was too afraid to say anything. How is that a safe learning environment?"

She shook her head, her voice cracking slightly.

"Then there was Margaret. She clearly doesn't want to precept anyone. She's impatient, annoyed with me all the time, or just jumps in and does everything before I even get a chance. It makes me so anxious coming to work. I feel like I'm not learning what I'm supposed to be learning."

"Yes, Natalie... I understand, but—"

"And another time, my preceptor didn't even know she was supposed to be with me until the shift started. That whole day, I just passed meds and turned patients. We barely spoke. Not a single conversation about what I needed to learn, what my goals were, or what I was still struggling with."

"Yes, but—"

"And then last week, with my sixth preceptor..." she paused, swallowing hard. "We had a patient fall. It was bad. He's going to need surgery, and his wife came in yesterday and blamed me to my face. Told me it was both our fault he's in agony. When I tried to talk to Clarisse about it, she told me I clearly wasn't cut out to be a nurse, that things happen, and to just get over it."

The Nurse Manager sighed and accepted the third resignation letter she had received since the beginning of the year.

"This isn't what I wanted when I chose nursing," Natalie said quietly. "I'm sorry, but I can't stay. Anyone in this profession who makes you feel like quitting isn't a good preceptor."

The Role of Preceptorship

Preceptorship is a structured relationship between an experienced nurse and a less experienced or novice nurse. Its goal is to develop clinical skills, competence, and confidence through an orientation period that typically spans several weeks or months. This role should not be confused with a mentor. A mentor is a trusted advisor who provides guidance, support, and knowledge to someone less experienced. Mentors can be formal or informal, their guidance are usually based on experience. Mentors use their wisdom when providing constructive feedback to their mentee.

The preceptor serves as a professional role model, demonstrating core responsibilities and standards of practice. In addition, they assess clinical competence and offer support, feedback, and guidance. To be effective, preceptors must cultivate strong interpersonal, teaching, and assessment skills (Hardie et al., 2022).

Preceptorship is a widely utilized framework in healthcare fields such as nursing, medicine, pharmacy, and allied health. It creates a one-on-one teaching and learning relationship that promotes professional development and real-time learning (Lofmark et al., 2012).

Preceptors play a crucial role in shaping a nurse's educational and clinical experience. During the final semester of nursing school, students are typically assigned a preceptor in a clinical setting. This "capstone" rotation allows students to apply classroom knowledge in real-world patient care under close supervision. Depending on school policy, the capstone usually lasts several weeks.

After graduation, new nurses are assigned a preceptor for at least three months. In some specialties such as Intensive Care or the specialized Operating Rooms, orientation may extend to six months or even longer depending of level of competency milestones reached by the preceptee. During this time, preceptors guide new nurses in developing essential skills, clinical knowledge, critical thinking, and professional etiquette.

It's important to note that nursing orientation is not exclusive to new graduates. Nurses transitioning from one specialty to another—for example, moving from Pediatrics to an adult Cardiovascular Intensive Care Unit—must also complete a tailored orientation, regardless of prior experience. During this period, they are treated as novices and require structured guidance from educators, clinicians, and preceptors to build competence. Through this process, preceptees are expected to grow more proficient and, over time, become experts. As they gain experience, they also develop stronger clinical reasoning and judgment skills (Benner et al., 2009).

Indicators of a Poorly Structured Precepting Program

Poorly designed or inconsistently applied preceptorship models can directly contribute to nursing turnover and staff shortages. Below are common indicators of weak or ineffective precepting programs:

1. Small Pool of Preceptors

A strong preceptorship program depends on a reliable group of qualified and willing preceptors. A limited pool forces educators to assign precepting duties to nurses who may lack specific training or genuine interest. This leads to inconsistency in teaching styles, fragmented orientation experiences, and a diminished sense of progress among preceptees. Without a standardized and adequately trained preceptor team, essential learning opportunities may be missed, delaying the development of autonomy and confidence in new nurses.

2. Inconsistent Preceptor Educational Standards

Each unit should have a designated Nurse Educator or Clinical Practice Leader responsible for overseeing orientation and preceptorship. In smaller hospitals, a single educator may cover multiple units or in some rare cases an entire service. Together with management, educators should define clear standards for preceptor training. This includes:

- Understanding each preceptor's teaching and learning style.
- Providing unit-specific clinical guidelines aligned with competency benchmarks.
- Offering regular skill refreshers to ensure that preceptors remain current on best practices.

Without clear and consistent educational standards, new nurses may receive conflicting or incomplete guidance from different preceptors.

3. Sink-or-Swim Approach

Some units rely heavily on task-based checklists, requiring preceptors to observe and sign off on completed duties. While this confirms procedural competence, it often fails to develop deeper clinical reasoning. Preceptees may be allowed to work independently before they are truly ready, unaware of their own knowledge gaps. This premature independence increases the risk of errors, especially during complex patient care situations.

4. Unsupportive Learning Environment

A toxic or unsupportive environment can negatively affect both students and new nurses. Clinical Professors may need to intervene when students face gossip, bullying, or belittling behavior from staff. New nurses often lack the confidence to speak up, especially in high-pressure clinical settings. These issues are even more damaging during orientation.

Preceptors have a duty to foster psychological safety and intervene in harmful situations. Dismissive behavior, exclusion, or gossip not only undermine learning but also contribute to burnout and high turnover.

One especially damaging behavior is known as "pilfered opportunity"—when experienced staff withhold bedside procedures or clinical experiences from preceptees. These hands-on skills, such as assisting with bronchoscopies, managing post-operative patients, or handling specialty medication drips, are critical for clinical growth. When preceptees are excluded from them, it limits their learning and damages morale.

5. Task-Based Learning vs. Reinforced Critical Thinking

Critical thinking involves reflective, reasoned decision-making in clinical situations. Its foundation includes recognizing problems, prioritizing actions, interpreting data, and evaluating outcomes. An effective preceptor not only teaches the "how" but also guides the "why" behind clinical decisions.

Strong preceptorship models integrate strategies that:

- Promote ongoing clinical assessment.
- Encourage curiosity and questions.
- Support decision-making through scenario-based reasoning.

Unfortunately, many units still emphasize speed and task completion over thought processes. While efficiency matters, task proficiency must be balanced with the development of sound clinical judgment—particularly when nurses face urgent or unpredictable patient needs. Without this balance, patient care quality and nurse confidence can suffer.

Actionable Steps to Improve Unit Precepting

1. Establish a Preceptor Recruitment and Retention Program

Develop an official program within the unit—or ideally across the entire service—to recruit and retain qualified preceptors. This program should offer well-defined incentives, such as financial compensation, clinical ladder advancement, or unit-based privileges. These incentives can be proposed by the Unit-Based Council or collaboratively created by the Unit Educator and Unit Leadership.

For example, some facilities provide preceptors with bonus paid time off, awarding twelve hours for each successful orientation. Another unit voted to offer preceptors a seniority preference when scheduling vacations, placing them just below the top five most senior nurses. These privileges acknowledge the time and dedication required to support new nurses effectively.

2. Evaluate Preceptors' Teaching Styles

Before orientation begins, take time to understand each preceptor's instructional preferences. This can be done informally through conversation or formally using tools like the Staffordshire Evaluation of Teaching Styles. When preceptors are aware of their teaching approach, they are better equipped to adapt to the learning styles of their preceptees, resulting in more effective teaching and improved outcomes.

3. Build Trust and Rapport

Trust forms the foundation of a successful precepting relationship. Preceptors should view themselves as approachable guides, ready to answer questions and provide feedback in alignment with unit education standards. When new nurses feel safe and supported, they are more likely to engage, grow, and succeed.

4. End-of-Shift Debriefing

Incorporate structured debriefs at the end of each shift. These debriefs should include reflection on:

- What went well
- What challenges arose
- Where knowledge gaps appeared
- What can be improved

This practice reinforces a collaborative learning culture. It helps normalize mistakes as part of the learning process and encourages open communication between preceptor and preceptee.

5. Be the Example

Leadership is not limited to designated roles. Every experienced nurse influences the learning environment. Nurses in leadership positions—or those viewed as senior—naturally become role models for behavior, professionalism, and patient care.

As John Wooden once said, "Being a role model is the most powerful form of educating." Nurses lead by example when they demonstrate respectful communication, patient-centered collaboration, and professionalism with both colleagues and patients.

Critical Point:

The way preceptors communicate, handle challenges, and interact with others teaches new nurses how to conduct themselves in professional settings. These everyday interactions are often more impactful than any policy manual or classroom session.

Teaching Strategies for a Better Orientation Experience

a. Direct Observation and Questioning

This is one of the most foundational teaching tools and should be used consistently. Preceptors observe preceptees during clinical tasks, then follow up with questions to assess their reasoning. If a response is inaccurate or incomplete, the preceptor can provide insight based on clinical experience or take time to explain best practices.

b. Weekly Readings

To help bridge knowledge gaps, Nurse Educators can assign weekly readings from peer-reviewed journals or recommend resources from the facility intranet. Websites like Medscape also provide accessible, evidence-based content to support clinical decision-making and lifelong learning.

c. Cheerleading (Positive Reinforcement)

Positive reinforcement strengthens confidence and reinforces growth. Preceptors should intentionally acknowledge moments when preceptees demonstrate progress—whether it's completing a task, showing critical thinking, or responding calmly in a clinical situation. This kind of encouragement not only supports retention but also contributes to a healthier, more collaborative work culture.

d. Timely Feedback

Effective preceptors offer regular, timely feedback. This can take place in end-of-shift conversations, scheduled evaluations, or quick check-ins throughout the day. Good feedback highlights strengths, identifies areas for growth, and offers clear next steps. The aim is always to coach, not to criticize.

e. Goal Setting

Encourage preceptees to set specific goals—daily or weekly—focused on skill development, knowledge retention, or even soft skills like patient interaction. Tangible goals help build a sense of progress and encourage autonomy. These goals can be revisited during end-of-shift debriefs and used to guide future learning.

f. Identifying Support Systems

New nurses should be introduced to the individuals and resources available to support them. This includes charge nurses, unit educators, nurse managers, and trusted colleagues. A successful orientation is not solely the responsibility of the preceptor—it depends on the collective support of the entire unit.

EVALUATION

Evaluation is a critical component of the orientation process. Since every healthcare system has its own policies and procedures for assessing clinical learning, skill development, and employee progress, those policies take precedence over the suggestions outlined here. This section offers recommended practices designed to strengthen the evaluation process, support a positive unit culture, and enhance nurse retention.

Preceptors should be thoroughly familiar with the healthcare system's, facility's, and unit's objectives for orientation. The following suggestions are focused on conducting evaluations in ways that foster strong working relationships, align with cultural values, and ultimately reduce staffing shortages.

1. Schedule evaluations in advance and provide a clear outline of expectations.

   Preceptees should receive an orientation roadmap that details the required skill sets, readings, and clinical standards they are expected to meet by each evaluation milestone. In units with a small preceptor pool, this outline can also guide substitute preceptors, helping maintain consistency and keeping orientation on track.

2. Hold a status-of-orientation meeting before the final evaluation.

   Regardless of how well the nurse manager, educator, or leader knows the preceptee, it should be standard practice to conduct a formal check-in meeting prior to the final evaluation. This meeting should include a review of the preceptee's progression, examples of improved competency, and goals they have achieved.

In short-staffed units, there is often pressure to expedite orientation so the new nurse can contribute to patient care as soon as possible. However, a rushed approach rarely inspires long-term commitment. Use this meeting to highlight the benefits of staying on the unit, discuss opportunities for growth, and invite the preceptee to take part in shaping the unit's culture. This is also a valuable opportunity to discuss a personalized development plan that aligns with both unit needs and the nurse's long-term career goals.

3. Agree on a feedback strategy before delivering evaluations.

   Before formal evaluations begin, the preceptor should determine how the preceptee prefers to receive feedback and agree on a delivery method with those participating in the evaluation. One effective approach at the midway point is the "feedback sandwich," which begins with positive comments, transitions into constructive feedback, and ends with another point of encouragement.

Another useful method is to focus on specific performance examples rather than personal characteristics. Reference documented goals, skills checklists, or facility-approved tracking tools to guide the conversation. This ensures the discussion stays professional and solution-focused. If concerns arise about unethical behavior or serious conduct issues, a different and more direct conversation is necessary.

Preceptees should seldom be surprised by an evaluation. If the preceptor has been offering consistent and constructive feedback throughout orientation, the formal evaluation should reinforce known strengths and areas for improvement.

4. Encourage self-evaluation before each meeting.

   While not always a formal requirement, self-directed reflection should be encouraged for all nurses, regardless of experience level. The ability to identify one's own strengths, mistakes, and knowledge gaps is essential to developing critical thinking skills.

Introducing self-evaluation during orientation helps normalize this reflective practice. It also reinforces the idea that accountability and continuous self-assessment are essential elements of professional nursing. Over time, this mindset shift can help elevate nursing culture and improve patient outcomes.

WORKING WITH THE DIFFICULT PRECEPTEE

At times, a preceptee may present ongoing challenges or show limited progress throughout orientation. The preceptor-preceptee dynamic is a relationship, and like any relationship, it can be affected by differences in personalities, learning styles, and values. Experienced preceptors are often skilled at navigating these difficulties, identifying the root causes, and working toward solutions.

Most commonly, challenges arise from performance concerns, poor communication, or a mismatch between the learner's style and the preceptor's approach. In other situations, the demands of the unit itself may overwhelm the preceptee. For example:

- In high-volume emergency departments, expecting a preceptee to manage six to eight patients can become especially difficult when staffing is limited. Frustration may build and spill over into the relationship, creating conflict that undermines learning. Temporarily reducing the patient load may help relieve the pressure and restore focus.

- In specialized Operating Rooms, long, complex procedures can lead to physical fatigue and mental exhaustion for preceptees who are not yet accustomed to extended hours and sustained concentration. Adjusting case assignments or limiting time spent in certain procedures can ease the burden and support better performance.

Often, what is labeled as "difficult" behavior stems from frustration, anxiety, feeling overwhelmed, or being unprepared. Other contributing factors may include personal distractions, health concerns, or inconsistencies in the orientation program. These challenges should be addressed through collaboration among the preceptor, management, and the unit's nurse educator.

The most powerful tool a preceptor has is a positive, supportive working relationship. Asking honest and compassionate questions can reveal underlying issues and guide potential interventions.

If the preceptor is unable to identify the source of the problem, they should involve management and the unit educator early in the process. Together, they can evaluate the situation and determine appropriate steps. If the preceptee continues to struggle despite targeted interventions, it may be necessary to consider transferring them to another unit or consider opportunities that might be a better fit in another specialty. In rare cases, separation from employment may be required.

While parting ways with a newly hired nurse is never easy, patient safety and care quality must remain the top priorities. Any consistent behavior or pattern that puts patients at risk cannot be ignored.

When preparing for a difficult conversation about a preceptee's future, it is important to:

- Clearly outline concerns as specific performance-related issues
- Reference relevant facility policies to provide structure and transparency
- Emphasize that decisions are based on documented actions, not personal judgments
- Keep the focus on ensuring the highest standard of care for patients

Nurse preceptors play a vital role in building strong, resilient nursing teams by coaching and mentoring the next generation of caregivers. When handled with clarity and compassion, this process becomes a foundation for a thriving unit culture.

Free Goodwill

Hello friend,

People who help others with zero expectation tend to experience higher levels of fulfillment. We are just at the half way point and I have a simple question for you...

Would you help someone you've never met, if it didn't cost you money, but you never got credit for it?

If so, I have an "ask" to make on behalf of someone you do not know. And likely, never will.

The goal of this book and our company RealNursingDynamics.com is helping nurses whether at the bedside or in the office, implement new tools that make our time on the units, easier to manage. If at the end of the book, you found some value, would you please take a brief moment to leave an honest review of the book and its contents? It will cost you zero dollars and will take less than 60 seconds.

Your review will help....

With developing better courses, better publications and better tools for others to use within the nursing profession.

If you are reading on kindle or an e-reader you can scroll to the bottom of the book, then swipe up and it will automatically prompt a review.

If you are on audible hit the three dots in the top right of your device, click rate and review.

Thank you from all of us at RealNursingDynamics.com, we take your time and attention with high regard.

Back to our regular scheduled programming.

N4

COMMITMENT

"The best time to plant a tree was 20 years ago.
The second best time is now."
– Chinese Proverb

04

N4

COMMITMENT

Xzavier has been a Registered Nurse for nine years at a 650-bed Level I trauma center. For the past six years, he has worked on a busy, 28-bed surgical step-down unit that handles a wide range of complex cases, including vascular, gastrointestinal, general surgery, and neurosurgery. The unit remains consistently full, with high-acuity patients and a steady workflow.

Xzavier is one of only three veteran nurses on the unit. Jaeda, who works days, has five years of experience, and Jayden, who works nights, has seven years. Since Xzavier joined the unit, three different nurse managers have come and gone. The manager who hired him resigned two weeks before her scheduled return from maternity leave.

Four and a half years ago, Xzavier began casually tracking the turnover rate of full-time nursing staff. What started as a personal project became something more significant when the number of departures reached 60. Realizing that he, Jaeda, and Jayden were now the last experienced nurses remaining, he recognized that change was necessary. It was no longer enough to hope that new hires would stay. There needed to be a system to retain newer nurses and foster a culture where they could see themselves growing, thriving, and eventually stepping into leadership roles.

Xzavier reached out to Jaeda and Jayden to reflect on the experiences that had helped them grow professionally. After gathering their insights and reflecting on his own journey, he presented leadership with a proposal for a new program. This initiative would promote the value and benefits of becoming a Nurse Liaison Mentor.

The Nurse Liaison Mentor Role

The title was created for this publication as a framework for veteran nurses, management and nurse educators to better understand the value of this informal position. Regardless of facility size, bed count, or patient acuity, most nursing units have at least one informal Nurse Liaison Mentor. These individuals consistently demonstrate several vital qualities:

- Advocating for both patients and staff during rounds, huddles, and interdisciplinary meetings
- Serving as a reliable resource when other nurses have questions about medications, interventions, or documentation
- Acting as an intermediary between frontline staff and leadership when needed
- Reinforcing unit culture and expectations through constructive, supportive feedback

- Informally mentoring newly independent nurses, especially those experiencing the "reality shock" that can last up to six months after orientation
- Offering deep unit-specific knowledge, often surpassing colleagues in situational awareness, even when total nursing experience is similar

Their presence can positively affect retention, outcomes, and morale. Xzavier's vision was to formalize this informal role, creating a program that would recognize, support, and develop Nurse Liaison Mentors. This would help preserve the culture of the unit and support its continued growth.

Actionable Steps to Develop Nurse Liaison Mentors

1. Advocate for and Promote Specialty Certification

a. Specialty certification expands clinical knowledge and is particularly impactful during the exam preparation process. Supporting continuing education and certification enhances job satisfaction and serves as a tool for attracting and retaining talented nurses. A culture of growth and development builds loyalty and reduces turnover.

b. Certification also increases clinical confidence by exposing nurses to the subtleties of their specialty. Since certification is voluntary, pursuing it demonstrates a nurse's commitment to high-quality care and professional development.

c. Continued education reduces the likelihood of clinical errors in medication administration, procedural interventions, and patient safety. It enhances clinical judgment and sharpens decision-making, especially in high-stress scenarios.

d. Achieving certification affirms a nurse's expertise to patients, colleagues, and providers. It also reflects the unit's dedication to excellence and signals leadership's investment in staff development.

2. Celebrate Loyalty

Recognition of tenure is a simple yet powerful way to boost morale and foster camaraderie. Acknowledging years of service cultivates pride and helps team members feel seen and valued.

One effective strategy is for the unit manager to schedule a one-on-one meeting 20 to 30 days before a nurse's work anniversary. This meeting can be used to reflect on the nurse's experiences, accomplishments, and aspirations. It also allows leadership to ask meaningful questions about how they can better support the nurse's personal and professional goals moving forward.

3. Role Model an Approachable Demeanor

Any successful working relationship depends on two key elements: trust and communication. Nurse Liaison Mentors should lead by example by modeling approachability and openness.

This means being open to staff approaching the Nurse Liaison for a conversation either in the present moment or another time during the shift that's more convenient. This accessibility, encourages trust, and signals that staffs are welcome to share constructive feedback about the unit or concerns in a positive, solution-focused manner.

By cultivating this approachable presence, Nurse Liaison Mentors promote transparency and help strengthen the overall unit culture. It also gives them opportunities to practice mentorship conversations and coaching techniques, preparing them to support others more effectively.

4. Prioritize Professional Development

Providing clear and accessible opportunities for professional growth is essential for engaging, retaining, and advancing nursing staff. Whether through continuing education, hands-on workshops, or formal mentorship programs, investing in the development of Nurse Liaison Mentors benefits both individual nurses and the broader team.

Nurse managers and educators should collaborate with veteran nurses to identify two or three personal and professional development goals. Together, they can set realistic timelines, outline the necessary steps, and determine how leadership will actively support their progress.

By fostering clinical expertise and aligning with long-term career aspirations, leadership creates an environment that supports deeper engagement, stronger loyalty, and greater job satisfaction. These qualities are essential for building and sustaining a high-performing unit.

N5

CAPABILITY

A leader without followers is just a man out taking a walk.
- John Boehner

05

N5
CAPABILITY

THE NURSE MANAGER PART ONE

The Nurse Manager role is one of the most demanding, if not *the* most demanding, positions in all of nursing. Nurse Managers lead their teams by setting a clear vision for the unit's progress toward clinical and operational excellence. They act as the chief change agents for their units, making critical decisions that shape the unit's culture, workflow, and overall success. Regardless of the unit's size or the number of staff members they oversee, the role can often feel daunting, and at times, nearly impossible to fulfill.

At its foundation, the Nurse Manager's responsibilities can be organized into what we'll call **The Core Four Responsibilities**. While some specialties may add or adjust responsibilities based on their specific needs, these core areas remain central to effective nursing leadership.

Team Management and Leadership

1. Nurse Managers serve as both the primary supervisors and clinical leaders of their units. They develop and uphold care standards specific to their patient population and services, providing direction to ensure these standards are consistently met. Their role is

crucial in overseeing daily patient care practices and ensuring clinical staff adhere to policies and guidelines.

In addition to operational oversight, Nurse Managers are heavily involved in mentorship, career development, and conflict resolution. By encouraging open dialogue and addressing tensions promptly, they help reduce toxicity and foster a healthier work environment. Their leadership in establishing a shared vision, balancing diverse perspectives, and creating a culture of support directly impacts the effectiveness and morale of the healthcare team.

2. Influencing Unit Culture

As discussed in *Nightingale 1: Shifting Culture*, while the Nurse Manager holds significant influence over the unit's operations, it is important to remember that the team itself is the culture. The manager shapes this culture by providing resources, setting clear expectations, and leading by example. However, it is the collective attitudes and behaviors of the staff that ultimately define the environment.

A successful Nurse Manager consistently works to maintain a positive, collaborative unit atmosphere. This means actively supporting team members, promoting transparent communication, addressing conflicts without delay, and routinely assessing the unit's overall morale and culture. When issues arise, effective managers make timely adjustments to keep the unit running smoothly and cohesively.

3. Managing Unit Staffing Needs

Staffing is one of the Nurse Manager's most immediate and ongoing responsibilities. Managers work closely with the in-house staffing coordinator to ensure every shift, whether four hours, eight hours, or more, is adequately staffed to meet patient care demands.

However, staffing can quickly become complex. Units experiencing crises or critical shortages often receive priority, leaving other services below optimal staffing levels. This can create frustration for managers and their teams. An added complication is unit acuity—the clinical intensity and complexity of the patient population. As acuity rises, so does the need for additional staffing to safely manage the workload.

As outlined previously on page 33, increased acuity refers to a higher number of clinically challenging patients who require more resources and staff support. Nurse Managers must remain agile, adjusting staffing plans as patient needs shift throughout the day and night.

4. Budget Oversight

Nurse Managers are responsible for drafting and managing their unit's annual budget. This includes tracking expenditures, ensuring costs stay within the allocated amount, and proactively identifying potential financial challenges.

Operational issues such as medical errors, insufficient training, high staff turnover, and gaps in professional development can quickly drain a unit's financial resources. Nurse Managers collaborate closely with administration and finance teams to address both major and minor budgetary concerns. Their ability to manage resources effectively has a direct impact on patient outcomes, staff retention, and overall unit performance.

Expectations, Standards and Patient Experience

1. Establishing and maintaining team member expectations

This includes ensuring that all nurses fully understand their roles, responsibilities, and the policies that govern their practice. To keep the unit aligned with healthcare regulations and accreditation standards, Nurse Managers set and reinforce performance benchmarks. These standards help the unit remain compliant, efficient, and clinically excellent.

2. Patient Safety

Nurse Managers play a central role in maintaining high standards of nursing care. They implement performance expectations based on National Patient Safety Goals, as well as facility-wide and unit-specific policies.

Managers are directly involved in reviewing performance evaluations, leading quality audits, and approving final performance sign-offs. They also analyze incident reports and provide individualized feedback to team members to prevent recurrence and promote safer outcomes for patients. Their consistent oversight helps reinforce a culture of accountability and continuous improvement.

3. Patient and Family Satisfaction

A patient's satisfaction is shaped by every interaction they have, from the moment they arrive at the facility to the time they are discharged. Nurse Managers work to ensure that this experience is positive, compassionate, and coordinated. One of the key tools used to assess this is the Hospital Consumer Assessment of Healthcare Providers and Systems (HCAHPS), a standardized survey administered after discharge that captures the patient's perspective of care. Nurse Managers use this and other tools to improve bedside communication, staff responsiveness, and overall patient experience.

They also promote strong interdisciplinary collaboration, ensuring that the needs of both patients and their families are consistently met across all touchpoints of care.

Recruitment and Retention

1. The Nurse Manager as Chief Recruiter

Nurse Managers are often at the forefront of recruitment efforts. Many use student clinical rotations as opportunities to identify high-potential candidates before graduation. Some establish formal partnerships with nursing schools to build recruitment pipelines, while others participate in job fairs hosted by the facility. Another strategic opportunity lies in converting travel nurses to permanent staff by creating a welcoming and supportive work culture that encourages them to stay long term.

2. Retention: Sustaining a Strong Team

Finding talented nurses is only half the battle; keeping them is just as critical. Nurse Managers influence retention by fostering a positive, empowering work environment where nurses feel valued and supported.

This includes:

- Building a culture of recognition and appreciation
- Creating opportunities for growth and advancement
- Promoting work-life balance and flexibility
- Encouraging open communication and feedback

When a nurse does choose to leave, the Nurse Manager can gain important insights through exit interviews and anonymous surveys, using this feedback to improve retention strategies moving forward.

3. Orientation and Continuous Learning

After a new nurse is hired, proper onboarding is essential. As explored in *Nightingale 3: Coaching (Precepting)*, orientation goes beyond paperwork; it's about fully integrating the nurse into the team and setting them up for long-term success. Precepting plays a key role in this process. Nurse Managers must ensure that each new hire is paired with a preceptor who fits their learning style and clinical needs. While the Unit Educator leads the technical and training aspects of orientation, the Nurse Manager is responsible for monitoring the overall effectiveness of the onboarding experience and stepping in when adjustments are needed. Successful orientation and continued learning are key ingredients in both short-term performance and long-term staff retention.

Collaboration and Coordination with Hospital Administration

1. Interdisciplinary Relationships

Nurse Managers must maintain positive, professional working relationships with a wide range of healthcare providers who contribute to patient care on the unit. These include:

- Attending Physicians
- Surgeons
- Respiratory Therapists
- Physical Therapists
- Social Workers
- Environmental Services Personnel
- Other Allied Health Professionals

Effective collaboration with these teams ensures that patient care remains comprehensive, seamless, and patient-centered.

2. The Bridge to Administration

Nurse Managers serve as the vital link between hospital administration and the nursing staff. A significant portion of their role involves attending administrative and organizational meetings, where they represent and advocate their unit's concerns, insights, and needs. Because they are fluent in both clinical nursing practice and administrative operations, Nurse Managers advocate for their teams while ensuring organizational objectives are met. What makes this position unique is that Managers can step into patient rooms to provide bedside care when needed, offering both leadership and firsthand support. Most Nurse Managers have experienced the pressures of short staffing, difficult work environments, and the challenges of mentoring new nurses. Their role requires a delicate balance between administrative duties, coaching responsibilities, and frontline supervisory tasks. Juggling these often-conflicting demands is one of the primary sources of frustration in the Nurse Manager role.

Why Do Nurse Managers Quit?

Recent national data highlights the growing strain on Nurse Managers:

According to the 2024 NSI Nursing Solutions Survey, 9.5% of Nurse Managers left their positions in 2023. Projections for 2024 estimate that 10.9% will leave, driven largely by the ongoing retirement of baby boomers. (NSI, 2024)

The 2024 AMN Healthcare Survey reported the top three challenges cited by Nurse Managers:

- 43% named recruitment and retention
- 32% identified staff burnout
- 32% cited labor shortages

The same survey revealed that 72% of Nurse Leaders reported experiencing burnout either sometimes, often, or always. (AMN, 2024)

Common burnout factors include:

- Excessive workload
- Inadequate staffing
- Limited leadership support
- Hostile or toxic work environments
- Poor work-life balance

While facilities typically provide formal training for the administrative functions of a Nurse Manager's role, the people-management skills – supporting, supervising, and maintaining a cohesive team – are often learned through experience. This creates an uneven preparation gap that contributes to frustration and turnover.

Guidelines for Enhancing Unit Culture and Team Support

To help Nurse Managers strengthen their leadership approach and shift their unit culture from survival mode to thriving mode, the following guidelines offer practical, incremental strategies. They focus on two core areas:

1. Maximizing Value During Floor Time

Most Nurse Managers can only devote about 20% of their working hours to direct unit presence due to administrative obligations. This limited time should be treated as a crucial opportunity to:

- Build personal rapport with staff
- Identify barriers to workflow efficiency
- Provide immediate coaching and recognition
- Address minor issues before they escalate

Maximizing the impact of floor time helps foster trust, morale, and team cohesion.

2. Promoting Unit Cohesiveness

A strong, united team culture reduces burnout, improves patient outcomes, and supports retention. This involves:

- Regularly engaging with team members to understand their concerns and experiences
- Acknowledging successes both big and small
- Facilitating open communication between nurses and interdisciplinary partners
- Reinforcing a culture of mutual respect and accountability

These strategies are most effective when implemented collaboratively with the Nurse Leaders and Charge Nurses the Nurse Manager supervises. Taking on these tasks alone can feel overwhelming, so gradual, consistent implementation — a few strategies at a time — will be key.

The Payoff: From Survival to Thriving

Meaningful, consistent leadership interventions may not yield immediate results, but over time they build a resilient, motivated, and high-functioning nursing team. The ultimate reward is transforming your unit culture from one of daily survival to sustainable, thriving success.

Build Relationships

Nurse Managers who want to foster stronger connections and build trust with their teams must be intentional about building relationships. Spending most of your time behind a desk, away from the unit, makes it nearly impossible to provide the resources and support your staff needs to be successful. To stay connected, Nurse Managers need to deliberately schedule time on the unit.

This can be a challenge, especially for managers overwhelmed by the growing stack of administrative responsibilities that land on their desks week after week. But what's the point of being on top of paperwork if the very staff you're meant to lead, support, and engage hardly see you? Visibility on the unit is non-negotiable.

1. Purposeful Leadership Rounding

Leadership rounds are brief, meaningful conversations between managers and staff designed to strengthen relationships. These rounds should be a regular, scheduled part of daily routines, not an afterthought. Their purpose is to build rapport, identify what's working well, gather suggestions for improvement, and decide on next steps to address concerns.

Key recommendations from a Leadership Rounding Toolkit:

- Know Your Purpose: Your main goal is to create a positive connection and build trust with each team member. Rounding is one of the most effective tools for ensuring staff feel heard, valued, and appreciated, while also gaining first-hand insight into what's working and what isn't from the people on the front lines.

- Be Consistent: Rounding must be a hardwired habit. Schedule it, announce it, and stick to it. Aim to round weekly, ensuring every employee is seen at least once a quarter. Be flexible, as staff work around the clock and every day presents different challenges. Find the time that works for them.
- Communicate the Why: Let staff know why leadership rounding matters and what they stand to gain from it. Be clear about their role in the process and how it benefits both them and the entire unit.
- Practice Active Listening: Use this time to truly listen. Don't just disseminate information — have purposeful, two-way conversations. Remember, staff often assume leadership already knows what's wrong. Asking them directly brings issues to the surface and invites them to be part of the solution.
- Document Key Takeaways: Keep a simple, efficient log of what you learn. It should take no more than five minutes to jot down notes, observations, and names of team members who deserve recognition. This record also helps you share insights with leadership teams and track progress.
- Follow Up and Follow Through: Turn what you hear into action. Start with achievable "quick wins" to show staff their voices matter. Share updates about what's been learned and what changes are being made as a result. (Apold, 2019)

2. Manager Huddles

In many units, the Charge Nurse leads the daily pre-shift huddle while the Manager remains in the office, particularly on night shifts. When possible, Nurse Managers should be present before the day shift huddle, as this is the one time both overnight and day shift teams are present.

These quick huddles are critical opportunities to communicate directly with staff on both shifts. They allow a brief conversation to take place, creating "situational awareness" about the complexities of the healthcare environment for that day. In addition, a huddle enables concerns to move through the proper channels to implement solutions more quickly and efficiently. (Schatz, 2022)

Equally important is how managers speak during these huddles. Every session is a chance to model the calm, honest, and optimistic leadership you want reflected in your team. And in units where huddles take place near patient care areas, remember to be mindful of what is said and how it's said, as patients and families may be within earshot.

3. Provide Recognition

With the support of your Unit-Based Council, find meaningful ways to recognize and celebrate your team. As Maya Angelou wisely said:

"People will forget what you said, people will forget what you did, but people will never forget how you made them feel."

Recognition fosters engagement and boosts morale. A simple, effective gesture is celebrating work anniversaries. Team members with 5, 10, or 15 years of service deeply appreciate acknowledgment of their dedication.

About 30 to 45 days before a team member's anniversary, schedule a one-on-one meeting. Use this time to discuss their professional goals, get feedback on changes within the unit, address any concerns or conflicts, and strengthen your relationship. Share some of your own experiences too. Building rapport is a two-way street.

Cultivate Trust

In any relationship, trust and communication are foundational. Without trust, Nurse Managers will struggle to influence positive change on their unit. This often results in increased turnover and staffing shortages.

Positive cultural shifts thrive on behaviors that build trust: being kind, transparent, consistent, and maintaining open lines of communication. When staff trust their Nurse Manager, change is easier to implement, turnover decreases, and managers can focus on preserving and improving the culture they've built.

Conversely, toxic behaviors, such as being dismissive, disengaged, disrespectful, or failing to follow through, quickly erode trust and damage team morale.

1. Open Door Policy

If your door isn't already open, it will be soon. Your staff will knock, often. Be proactive about creating an Open Door Policy that promotes trust and transparency.

- Improved Communication: Let your team know that when your door is open, even if you're working, you're available to listen. Staff often hesitate to approach managers for fear of being a bother. An open door sends a message that their voice matters.
- Increased Trust: When staff feel safe approaching leadership with concerns, ideas, or personal matters, it fosters a culture of openness and trust. It also helps managers address problems early, before they escalate.
- Confidentiality: Depending on your facility's policies, reassure staff that conversations will remain confidential. Knowing their concerns are handled respectfully and discreetly empowers them to speak up.

2. Be Transparent

Nursing consistently ranks as the most trusted profession, and rightfully so. Patients expect honesty, and so do staff. Frustration often stems from not understanding the "why" behind decisions.

Take the time to explain what's happening within the organization and how those decisions affect the unit. While some changes may still be difficult to accept, clarity makes them easier to process.

- Communicate Openly and Honestly: Make it a priority to be truthful and direct, even when the news is difficult. Understand that reactions may vary. Some staff will appreciate the honesty while others may resist, especially during unit cultural shifts. Stay consistent. Over time, resistance diminishes.

- Acknowledge Mistakes: A 2010 study (Carroll, 2014) revealed that nurses and pharmacists, despite fearing blame, were more likely than physicians to report errors, regardless of severity. As a leader, be transparent about your own mistakes. Use them as teaching moments. This models the professionalism and accountability you expect from your team. For new managers, giving yourself grace is crucial. Leadership comes with a steep learning curve.

3. Be Consistent in Your Follow-Up

Your actions must align with your words. Deliver information clearly and consistently across your team.

Use notes from leadership rounds, feedback from open-door conversations, and your own observations to determine which priorities to address and when. Share progress updates regularly, whether it's about new initiatives, operational changes, or team concerns. Visible, consistent follow-through is one of the fastest ways to build and sustain trust.

Set Unit-Based Goals

Team synergy and interdependence are essential for delivering high-quality, safe patient care. Each year, nursing units adopt National Patient Safety Goals targeting specific areas for improvement. Facilities also track internal goals and metrics to identify opportunities for progress within individual units. One of the Core Four responsibilities for Nurse Managers is setting staff expectations. Establishing unit-based goals is a powerful tool to foster teamwork, accountability, and improved outcomes.

How to Set Effective Unit-Based Goals

a. Identify a Pain Point

Start by identifying a unit issue that hinders care delivery. Commonexamplesinclude:

- Inconsistent unit teamwork leading to poor quality patient care
- Lack of supplies, broken equipment, or disorganized rooms and unit spaces
- Poor interdisciplinary collaboration that causes miscommunication, frustration, and decreased trust

b. Facilitate Conversations During Huddles

Begin addressing these issues during unit huddles. Explain how they impede patient care and increase risk, using peer-reviewed data and unit policies to support your points. Reinforce your belief in the team's ability to overcome these challenges and continue delivering excellent care.

c. Ensure Resources Are in Place

Gather feedback from team members or survey the unit to identify barriers:

- Are scanners broken or missing in several rooms?

- Is there a better system that could be used to organize unit supplies and equipment?
- What communication or accountability issues are obstructing interdisciplinary cohesion?

Clarify these obstacles before setting any expectations.

d. Set the Unit Goal and Consistently Communicate It

As discussed earlier, use SMART Goals. For example:

"The unit medication scan rate will be a minimum of 98% within three months from today."

Announce the goal consistently — during manager huddles, in unit-wide emails, and on a visible poster board that includes the goal, its importance, and the next review date.

During leadership rounds, hold informal check-ins. Ask team members how the new scanners are functioning, what improvements could be made, and whether there is any resistance to the changes.

e. Measure, Report, and Recognize

Track both progress and obstacles. Celebrate small wins to build momentum, and turn setbacks into learning opportunities.

For areas that fall short, identify the root causes and hold brief, supportive coaching sessions with the team members involved. These sessions can also be led by Nurse Liaisons or Unit Educators.

f. Provide Recognition and Reinforce Standards

Make it clear that the new standard is not temporary – it is the permanent standard.

At year's end, compile the unit's achievements and display them in a high-traffic staff area such as the break room, multipurpose room, or Unit-Based Council meeting room. This visual reminder of collective progress reinforces shared accountability and pride.

Navigating the Night Shift

Healthcare is unique in its need for continuous, 24-hour care. There's a saying in the profession: "Nursing is a 24-hour, never-ending job," and it holds true. The standards and expectations for patient care during the day and evening apply just as much overnight.

However, night shifts present unique challenges – sleep deprivation, alarm fatigue, reduced resources, and the absence of many specialty teams. These factors can lead to feelings of isolation, disengagement, and the long-standing perception that "nobody cares about the night shift."

Nurse Managers must take deliberate steps to maintain team cohesion, morale, and accountability across all shifts. Overnight staff deserve to be fully engaged in unit goals and supported in their roles, just like their daytime counterparts.

Night Shift Leadership Toolbox: Action Items & Rationales

1. Involve Night Shift in Unit Decisions

Use the night shift facilitator from the Unit-Based Council to relay leadership updates and gather feedback both ways.

Before launching any new initiative, make sure night shift staff are informed through the most effective channel for your unit — whether that's email, an approved group messaging app, or a secure Electronic Medical Record-based chat platform.

2. Develop a Clear Communication Plan

Day shift staff typically benefit from direct access to managers through open-door policies and in-person rounding.

Create a communication protocol specifically for night shift. Define how and when they can reach you after hours for urgent matters, while maintaining respect for your off-duty hours.

3. Ensure Leadership Visibility

Plan for yourself or a designated leadership team member to work part of a night shift occasionally. This could be one full shift per month or a shorter early morning overlap between 5 AM and 7 AM.

Use that time to complete leadership rounds, listen to concerns, identify resource needs, discuss ongoing goals, and build trust with overnight staff.

4. Review Staffing Coverage Before Leaving

Before ending your shift, take a moment to double-check the assignment sheet and confirm that the night shift is properly staffed.

If you notice any issues, connect with the house supervisor or staffing coordinator.

Even if you can't fix the problem immediately, this step shows the night team that leadership is attentive to their workload and concerned about patient safety.

5. Address Conflict Promptly and Fairly

Tension between day and night shift teams often arises from miscommunication or perceived imbalance. When conflict surfaces:

- Meet with both individuals or teams to understand their perspectives
- Determine if the issue is an isolated incident or a broader pattern
- Choose an appropriate resolution based on the nature and impact of the situation

6. Regularly Assess Night Shift Workload

Make it a point to continually evaluate the workload of night shift staff. Gather feedback about equipment or process limitations that affect patient care.

Bring in support from the Unit-Based Council, Nurse Educators, and provider partners to troubleshoot and improve working conditions for night staff.

THE NURSE MANAGER PART TWO

Employee Engagement

The concept of employee engagement was introduced in 1990 by organizational behavior professor William A. Kahn in his article *"Psychological Conditions of Personal Engagement and Disengagement at Work."* Kahn's article was the first to explore this concept in management theory. He defined employee engagement as "the use of an employee's identity in their work role." In essence, he described how employees express parts of their identity through their performance at work.

Employee engagement remains one of the leading frameworks for improving workplace productivity and increasing staff retention. However, it is sometimes misunderstood, and its application as a framework can be contentious. At its core, employee engagement is the emotional commitment an employee has to their work, their team's goals, and their organization's mission. Simply put, it's about the emotional connection employees feel toward their company.

What Employee Engagement Is Not

It is *not* about making sure your employee is happy.

A nurse may be happy when patient acuity is low or when they're working alongside close friends – but that doesn't necessarily make them more productive. Happiness is fleeting and subjective.

It is *not* about food as a reward.

Across the country, nursing units rely on food-based gestures — from pizza parties to ice cream socials — to recognize milestones like successful Joint Commission visits or weeks without patient falls. While these are appreciated, they are momentary rewards. They do not build emotional connection or long-term commitment.

What the Numbers Say

PRC, a national healthcare market research company, conducted a 2023 Nursing Engagement Report surveying 1,923 RNs from 37 hospitals across the United States. Nurses answered 34 questions on nurse quality indicators, engagement, burnout, and retention. Key findings include:

- 45.1% of nurses reported being "fully engaged," 40.5% "engaged," and 14.4% "unengaged."
- Among unengaged nurses, 41.9% reported burnout, compared to 7.6% of fully engaged and 14.9% of engaged nurses.
- Only 50.7% of unengaged nurses intended to stay with their organization for at least two more years, compared to over 80% of engaged and fully engaged nurses.
- Engagement levels varied by generation, shift time, and practice setting. Millennial and night-shift nurses reported lower engagement rates. (King & Bradley, 2023)

By comparison, the Gallup 2024 *State of the Workplace* Report found that across all industries:

- 23% of American workers are engaged
- 62% are not engaged
- 15% are actively disengaged. (Gallup, 2024)

Recognizing Types of Employee Engagement

Through observation, feedback, and performance reviews, Nurse Managers often see three common categories of engagement:

1. **Highly Engaged**

   These nurses are productive, eager to contribute, and committed to the team long-term. Their traits are similar to those of a Nurse Liaison Mentor, discussed in *Nightingale 4: Commitment*.

2. **Moderately Engaged**

   These nurses are well-liked by peers and generally content with their job but may feel stagnant. They rarely seek out additional responsibilities.

3. **Disengaged**

   These team members often do the bare minimum. They may frequently voice goals unrelated to unit priorities and leave once personal goals are met. They tend to lack emotional connection to the team or organization — and if left unchecked, they can influence others to disengage as well. This often contributes to unit toxicity.

What Drives Nursing Engagement

According to the 2023 Nurse Engagement Survey, three primary drivers improve engagement:

Autonomy

Nurses who feel included in decision-making and believe their opinions matter are more engaged.

- Support Unit-Based Councils
- Encourage and fund specialty certification opportunities

Nurse-to-Nurse Teamwork and Collaboration

Nurses embedded in a supportive peer network are more engaged.

- Invest in relationship-building and accountability coaching as described in *Nightingale 1: Culture*

Leadership Access and Responsiveness

Trust in leadership and easy access to managers increase engagement.

- Maintain an Open Door Policy
- Conduct regular Leadership Rounds and annual professional development meetings
- Periodic night shift coverage improves perceptions of manager accessibility

Manage Your Bandwidth

Stress management begins with self-awareness. Recognizing your own emotional responses, understanding how they influence your behavior, and developing healthier coping strategies are essential to preserving your mental bandwidth.

Bandwidth refers to the personal energy we have for responsibilities each day. Work-related stress can reduce engagement and strain home life. Conversely, personal preoccupations can lead to distraction and poor work performance.

As Miyata (2015) noted, "The poor health of nurse managers indirectly and negatively affects their staff's health." Managers cannot perform at high levels without safeguarding their own well-being.

Self-Management Strategies

1. Self-Reflection

   A seasoned nurse might remember a handful of medication errors over thousands of doses. Similarly, nurse managers must reflect not only on challenges but also on what went well each day. Before leaving work, take a moment to assess what worked, what didn't, and how to grow from it.

2. Self-Awareness

   Recognize how your tone, body language, and reactions affect others. Identify your strengths — humor, empathy, problem-solving — and intentionally lead with them. This builds trust and camaraderie.

3. Personal Goal Setting

   Amid the demands of the job, don't lose sight of your own ambitions. Set SMART goals (Specific, Measurable, Achievable, Relevant, Time-bound) to stay focused. Break larger objectives into manageable steps with timelines and checkpoints. Post them where you'll see them daily — on your phone lock screen, desktop background, or workstation.

4. Self-Reward

   Accomplishments often go unacknowledged in leadership roles. Celebrate your wins — big or small. Book a massage, dine at your favorite restaurant, or plan a post-project gathering with peers. Recognition starts with you.

5. Self-Correcting Feedback (Self-Punishment)

   This entails positive honesty — reframing failures and unproductive actions in a way that helps reshape future behavior (Goldsby, 2020). Mistakes happen. What matters is how you respond. We tend to allow failures to occupy significant space in our thoughts, even when that brings no real benefit. Use failure as an opportunity to learn, grow, and reframe. As a role model, the grace and resilience you demonstrate after setbacks will shape your team's culture.

Keep What You've Built

The time, energy, and effort it takes to build a strong team and address staffing shortages is no small feat. A Nurse Manager must stay vigilant, committed to protecting the trust, culture, and standards they've worked hard to establish. The final two leadership responsibilities are essential for increasing the capability of your nursing team are recruitment and retention.

Improved Hiring Practices

Two important practices can improve your chances of bringing the right people on board: an enhanced shadow experience and a performance-based interview process.

Improved Shadow Experience

Depending on facility processes, the Nurse Manager may receive resumes directly or through the recruitment or staffing office, which screens candidates before forwarding them. This is typically followed by a phone or in-person interview, and sometimes a four-hour shadow shift where the candidate observes a working nurse and is interviewed afterward.

When used intentionally, the shadow experience becomes an invaluable tool for identifying candidates who are a good fit. To get the most out of it:

1. Select the Right Preceptor

   Choose the nurse who will be shadowed in advance. Provide clear guidance on the candidate qualities and behaviors to observe. This engages existing staff in team building and avoids the stress of last-minute assignments. Also, notify the rest of the team during huddle so they are aware and can engage with the candidate meaningfully.

2. Assign Strong Role Models

   Whenever possible, pair candidates with nurses who are known for their professionalism, strong work ethic, and positive attitude. Avoid assigning randomly. If the nurse is disengaged or unwilling, it can reflect poorly on the unit. Staffing shortages or poor planning should not compromise this step.

3. Set Clear Expectations

   Before the shadow shift begins, explain to the assigned nurse what is expected of them. Reinforce that their behavior should reflect the unit's standards of professionalism, collaboration, and bedside care. The goal is for the candidate to experience the kind of environment they would be joining.

4. Create a Two-Way Feedback Loop

   After the shadow shift, collect feedback from both the candidate and the precepting nurse. Ask the candidate: *What did you enjoy about your time here? What challenges did you notice?* Ask the nurse: *What strengths did you observe? Any concerns?*

5. Use these insights to improve both the candidate experience and your team culture.

Performance-Based Interviewing (PBI)

The traditional interview model often relies on hypothetical, situational questions like:

- What are your strengths and weaknesses?

- Where do you see yourself in five years?
- How important is teamwork to you?

While common, these types of questions rarely reveal how a person performs under pressure or navigates real challenges.

Performance-Based Interviewing (PBI) is an evidence-based method of interviewing staff. It involves giving candidates scenarios to assess their skills or asking open-ended questions about how they have managed specific situations in previous roles. The focus is on how a candidate performed in the past, the actions they took, and the outcomes of their decisions (Sherman, 2019).

The Nurse Manager should ask candidates to describe specific situations, followed by at least two follow-up questions to gain deeper insight. For example:

Critical Thinking

Tell me about a time you faced a problem with no ideal solution and potentially negative outcomes.

1. How did you decide what to do, and what was the result?
2. What was the biggest takeaway from that experience?

Patient Education

Describe a discharge situation where you had to educate a patient about something you weren't completely familiar with.

1. What two resources did you use to prepare?
2. How did you confirm everyone understood?

Patient Safety

Share a time you witnessed a safety issue caused by a patient's visitor.

1. How did you address it with the visitor?
2. What did you do to prevent it from happening again?

Communication

Tell me about a time you had to work with a difficult co-worker.

1. What was the hardest part about working with them?
2. How have your interactions with challenging coworkers changed since then?

Conflict Resolution

Was there a time you had to talk to an upset patient about an aspect of their care that you weren't responsible for? *Examples might include meal delivery, discharge medication orders, or a shift in plan of care.*

1. How did you respond to help decrease their anger or frustration?
2. What were your action steps to resolving the issues?

Developing these types of scenario-based questions can be a collaborative effort. Involve your Unit-Based Council, Assistant Nurse Managers, or Unit Educator. The questions should focus on identifying the key characteristics that best align with and enhance your workplace culture.

Retention: Keeping Good People

Nursing retention remains a significant challenge for many reasons. Baby Boomers who delayed retirement during the COVID-19 pandemic are now beginning to leave the workforce. By 2030, this trend will intensify as they reach the minimum retirement age for their generation.

At the same time, newer generations of nurses – particularly Gen Z – bring a different mindset to the profession. If a workplace does not align with their values, they are more likely to leave in search of better opportunities.

Two essential retention tools for Nurse Managers are exit interviews and employee surveys.

Exit Interviews

Exit interviews offer a valuable, candid look at your team's culture and management practices. Departing employees may feel freer to speak openly about their experiences without fear of repercussions.

The main goals of an exit interview are to:

- Learn where the unit can improve
- Ensure the employee leaves on a positive note
- Explore whether there is an opportunity to retain them under new circumstances (when appropriate) (Frase-Blunt, 2004).

Important guidelines:

a) Exit interviews should be reserved for voluntary separations. Issues raised by layoffs or terminations for cause require a different approach (Frase-Blunt, 2004).

b) Follow your facility's policies on whether HR or Nurse Managers conduct the interview.

c) Frame the interview as an opportunity to help the unit grow and improve.

d) The interview can be conducted either formally or informally. The goal is to obtain honest insights — even when the feedback is difficult — in order to better serve your team moving forward.

Actionable steps:

1. Make Exit Interviews an Expectation

   Let staff know from the beginning that their feedback matters — including when they decide to leave. Normalizing the process shows that the organization values learning from every experience.

2. Explain the Purpose

   Clarify that the goal of the interview is to improve the work environment for both current and future employees. Framing it as a constructive step helps ease discomfort.

3. Use a Thoughtful Questionnaire

   Prepare a set of written questions covering unit culture, leadership support, highlights of their experience, and areas for improvement. This gives departing staff time to reflect and helps guide the conversation productively.

4. Reassure Confidentiality

Recognize that some employees may worry about burning bridges, especially if they've formed close bonds with managers or peers. Reassure them that their feedback will be handled with discretion and respect.

5. Separate Ego from Feedback

   If staff critique management or leadership, don't take it personally. If it's difficult to remain neutral, consider assigning the interview to a third party. Objective listening ensures better insights.

6. Look Ahead, Not Just Back

   Exit interviews reflect the past, but their true value lies in shaping the future.

   - Analyze feedback to identify recurring patterns.
   - Organize findings by theme and regularly review them with your leadership team.
   - Focus on lessons learned and actionable improvements.

Unit Surveys

Surveys are an excellent way to gather continuous feedback on staff satisfaction and to spot opportunities for growth. Tools like SurveyMonkey and SurveySparrow offer customizable, user-friendly platforms.

Surveys can be comprehensive (used annually or semi-annually) or short and targeted — such as pulse surveys conducted before retreats, policy updates, or educational programs. Pulse surveys are especially valuable for quickly gauging morale and team sentiment on specific topics.

Steps for Effective Survey Implementation:

1. Identify Clear Goals

   Decide exactly what you want to learn. Are you evaluating staff morale, leadership effectiveness, or workflow bottlenecks?

2. Choose the Right Audience

   Consider whether to survey only nurses or include support staff such as techs, secretaries, and ancillary personnel.

3. Communicate the Purpose

   Let participants know why their input matters, how the data will be used, and that their responses will remain confidential.

4. Set a Realistic Timeline, Then Distribute

   Provide a clear deadline and ensure easy access to the survey. Distribute links via email or internal portals, or post QR codes on unit bulletin boards. As a backup, paper surveys can be used with a secure drop box for anonymous submissions. Keep in mind that tracking completion is easier with digital tools.

5. Collect and Analyze the Data

   Track participation rates and follow up with non-respondents as needed. Analyze the results to identify trends, recurring issues, and areas of concern. Use the findings to shape interventions that align with your unit goals.

6. Create an Action Plan

   Assign clear responsibilities for implementing changes. Share results and plans with staff so they can see how their feedback leads to action. Distribute the workload among the management team to ensure consistent follow-through.

"Successful leaders are good planners who understand that the building blocks need to be in place for initiatives to succeed. Leadership is critical at every stage of the change process. Managers need to implement tools to measure our progress. Nurse leaders sometimes complain about lack of staff compliance, yet the problem is that we don't build in mechanisms to hardwire changes into practice." (Sherman, 2019)

Nurse Managers have the power to transform their units. When applied consistently, the strategies outlined here — combined with thoughtful planning and a commitment to growth — provide the tools to develop and support a team that thrives. The results speak for themselves: increased job satisfaction, reduced staffing shortages, and better patient outcomes.

N6

CONTINUITY

If anything is certain, it is that change is certain.
- Philip Crosby

N6
CONTINUITY

Continuity can carry different meanings depending on the context, but generally refers to something that is uninterrupted, consistent, and dependable over time. In nursing, continuity refers specifically to the coordinated care a patient receives throughout their stay — from admission to discharge. This care may be provided by one healthcare professional or by a team working together to ensure seamless support.

Continuity of the Unit focuses on deliberately building unit guidelines, roles, and policies that promote teamwork and sustain high-quality care, even as staff members transition in and out. The goal is to design effective transition plans and operational structures that uphold patient care standards and keep the unit functioning smoothly. Anticipating and addressing disruptions proactively also helps reduce factors contributing to staffing shortages or workflow breakdowns.

BOOM LOOP

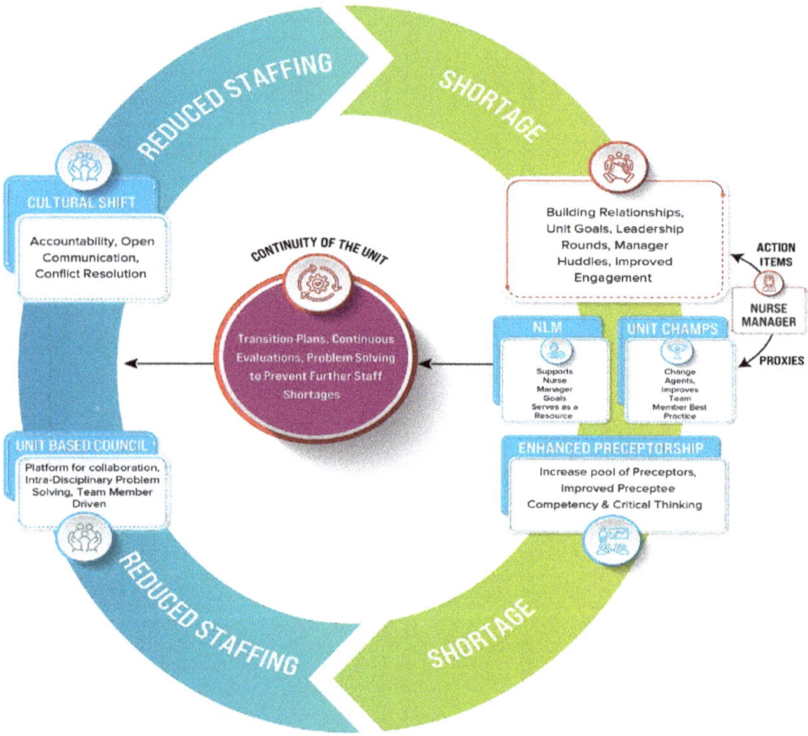

The Boom Loop is a performance dashboard illustrating continuous improvement processes that help stakeholders identify how they can strengthen their role in reducing staffing shortages.

1. Shifting Unit Culture

Reducing toxicity and incivility — two major drivers of burnout and turnover — requires fostering a healthier, more supportive work environment. This shift encourages nurses to take responsibility for their behaviors and relationships, reinforcing mutual respect. A positive unit culture not only boosts morale and retention but also directly enhances patient care.

2. Embracing the Unit-Based Council (UBC)

The UBC supports collaboration through a shared governance model. By participating, nurses gain a voice in decision-making, take ownership of initiatives, and hold one another accountable. This alignment of organizational goals, leadership priorities, and frontline expertise leads to higher satisfaction, stronger retention, and improved outcomes.

3. Enhancing Coaching and Preceptorship

A strong onboarding process ensures that both new graduates and experienced hires gain essential unit knowledge and clinical confidence. Structured, supportive orientation strengthens nurse readiness and integration, improving satisfaction and long-term performance.

4. Creating Growth Opportunities for Experienced Nurses

Experienced nurses should be given meaningful leadership and mentorship roles. Assigning them as Nurse

Liaison Mentors acknowledges their value and uses their strengths to support newer staff. These mentors also help lighten the leadership load by acting as reliable, peer-based resources.

5. Strengthening Nurse Management

Effective nurse managers are critical to unit stability. Their leadership drives staff engagement, operational success, and patient care outcomes. Investing in their development is essential to sustaining a well-functioning unit.

6. Sustaining Unit Continuity

Continuity means having structured transition plans, including clear leadership succession within the UBC and designating Unit Champions. These roles provide operational stability and keep improvement initiatives moving forward despite staff changes.

Continuity of the Unit-Based Council (UBC)

Preparation

Before the departure of key UBC members like the Chair, Co-Chair, or facilitators, a transition plan should be in place. This includes identifying successors and updating recruitment efforts. Recruitment should spotlight the council's achievements and explain how new members can shape its future. This stage is about building awareness and preparing staff for upcoming changes.

Planning

The plan must define when and how new members will be introduced to the UBC's problem-solving model.

Shadowing current facilitators, interdisciplinary partners, or leadership offers valuable exposure. At the same time, responsibilities may need to be reassigned based on evolving unit needs.

Communication

Consistent, open communication throughout the transition is crucial. Share timely updates about UBC changes, member expectations, and start dates with the entire unit, including interdisciplinary staff. Keep everyone informed to maintain engagement and continuity.

Implementation and Support

Nurse managers, educators, and UBC leaders should monitor new member progress and maintain active support. Allow time for adjustment and schedule regular check-ins. After early UBC meetings, collect feedback to identify growth areas and reinforce a positive, supportive environment.

Unit Champions

When implemented strategically, nurse educators and nurse managers can reduce staffing shortages and improve quality of care by leveraging the strengths of Unit Champions. A Unit Champion is a nurse who demonstrates enthusiasm for learning, educating peers and patients, or developing leadership skills. Champions act as change agents in a variety of roles: educator, facilitator, mentor, leader, policy developer, and evaluator, all in support of best practice guidelines (White, 2011).

Unit Champions provide targeted education to both

patients and colleagues. In fast-paced clinical settings, nurses frequently turn to trusted peers for real-time guidance. Appointing champions as reliable resources fosters trust and teamwork, enhances unit cohesion, and helps reduce nursing turnover.

Actionable Steps for Developing Unit Champions

Recruitment and Training

1. **Communicate the Purpose and Benefits**

   Introduce the Unit Champion role clearly. Explain its purpose, the required training, available resources, and any associated incentives. Share the opportunity during unit huddles, display flyers in high-traffic areas, and send follow-up emails to reinforce interest.

2. **Identify Talent During Evaluations**

   Use annual evaluations to highlight nurses' individual strengths and discuss how becoming a champion can enhance patient care and support the nurse's own growth.

3. **Engage Informally**

   Listen for interest during casual conversations and observe staff interactions. Nurses who express a desire to grow or who naturally exhibit leadership behaviors may be excellent candidates.

4. **Interdisciplinary Collaboration**

   Pair each Unit Champion with a corresponding interdisciplinary team for mentorship and support.

For example, a Wound and Skin Care Champion could collaborate with the facility's Wound, Ostomy, and Continence Nurses (WOCN). If no such team exists, consider forming a small committee with qualified clinicians.

5. **Structure of Training**

a. Shadowing Opportunities

Arrange shadowing sessions with interdisciplinary partners. These sessions can take place during regular shifts or as approved overtime and should be hands-on and practical.

b. Educational Resources

Provide access to reliable materials in both physical and digital formats. These should be easy to locate — in-unit folders, shared drives, or the facility intranet.

c. Documentation Audits

Train champions to audit documentation effectively. Encourage them to highlight both areas needing improvement and examples of outstanding work to share as models with the team.

Develop Goals and Expectations

Unit Champions will continue fulfilling their regular duties while taking on new responsibilities. Establish clear expectations to support their success, such as:

1. **Promote Best Practices**

   Educate peers about current best practice guidelines using both formal presentations and informal conversations. Serve as a reliable, approachable resource (White, 2011).

2. **Model Best Practice**

   Master the content first, then demonstrate consistent use of best practice standards during bedside care. Lead by example to reinforce learning.

3. **Monitor Implementation**

   Track progress and share updates by presenting audit results during huddles, sending periodic emails, or using visual displays in shared spaces.

4. **Host Clinical Workshops**

   Work with the nurse educator and interdisciplinary partners to organize focused skills workshops that address unit needs and build clinical confidence.

Professional Organization Membership

Encourage all Unit Champions to join a professional nursing organization. When possible, managers or educators should cover membership fees. These organizations offer numerous benefits: continuing education, discounted certification exams, lower conference registration costs, and subscriptions to peer-reviewed journals (Cline, 2019).

With more than 300 professional nursing organizations in the United States – many focused on specific specialties – participation sends a clear message that professional development is supported and celebrated across the unit.

Continuity of the Position

When a Unit Champion steps down or transfers off the unit, having a clear succession plan is essential to maintaining continuity.

- **Preceptorship**

  Once a replacement is identified, the outgoing champion should actively train the incoming one. Whenever possible, schedules should be adjusted to allow for dedicated one-on-one time. Expecting someone to train while simultaneously managing a patient load compromises the quality of training and should be avoided.

- **Resource Orientation**

  The new champion must be fully oriented on how to access all relevant resources – including projects, educational materials, shared drive content, and unit-specific tools. If the unit hosts skills fairs, informal refreshers, or rotates clinical education posters, these processes and tools must be introduced as part of onboarding.

FINAL THOUGHTS

FINAL THOUGHTS

The Nightingale 6 is not a quick fix or one-time initiative. It is a sustained, evolving process that demands consistency, proper support, and a shared commitment.

Cultural transformation on a unit begins with accountability. Addressing incivility and toxic behaviors head-on empowers nurses to take ownership of their interpersonal conduct, fostering a respectful and collaborative environment. This shift not only improves the work experience but also enhances patient outcomes and retention.

The Unit-Based Council (UBC) plays a foundational role in this cultural transformation. Through shared governance, nurses are given a meaningful voice in shaping their unit's future. This structure promotes team-based collaboration, cultivates autonomy, and strengthens the alignment between frontline expertise and organizational goals.

Another pillar of sustainable improvement is a strong onboarding process. Through robust coaching and preceptorship, new or transferring nurses are equipped with the clinical confidence and unit-specific knowledge they need to thrive. As nurses gain experience, they must be given opportunities to grow. Elevating experienced nurses into Nurse Liaison Mentor roles acknowledges their contributions while extending their impact across the unit.

Nurse Managers are the linchpins of this entire process. Through authentic relationships, consistent engagement, and visible leadership, they build the trust and structure needed for continuity and success. Their ability to lead through change, nurture team strengths, and protect the culture they help establish directly impacts staffing stability.

Continuity means planning ahead. Whether a council member rotates off or a Unit Champion steps down, smooth transitions are essential. A well-supported Unit Champion program ensures that clinical excellence, mentorship, and leadership remain embedded in the daily life of the unit — bolstering peer support and strengthening patient care.

When applied consistently, the Nightingale 6 frameworks produce real, measurable progress. Small actions, taken each day, accumulate into lasting change. This approach keeps the focus exactly where it belongs — on patient outcomes. That is how nursing continues to earn and uphold its title as the most trusted profession in healthcare.

Together, by showing up, staying committed, and solving problems as a team, we can — and will — reduce staffing shortages.

> *"Nursing is a progressive art such that to stand still is to go backward."*
> ***— Florence Nightingale***

One More thing...

I am grateful for your time and attention. You could have given it to anything and you chose to invest your invaluable time with me.

From the bottom of my heart, Thanks!

- Gary

As a small token of my appreciation you can head to RealNursingDynamics.com and click on Products. The link will provide a ***free*** *gift from me to you.*

Our Mission:

To reduce nurse staffing shortages by transforming the way hospitals and healthcare systems onboard and retain nurses—through evidence-based preceptor program enhancement and equipping Nurse Managers with the skills to build resilient, high-performing teams.

Our Offerings:

Preceptor Program Audits and Optimization

Nurse Manager Online Courses

a. Empowering Nurse Managers to build resilient Teams
b. Nurse Manager toolkit for improving and implementing leadership rounds

Unit Specific Customized Consulting Services

Workshops and Speaking Engagements

Publications

If any of this peaks your interest we would love to meet you and hear about your challenges and see if we can help.

REFERENCES

REFERENCES

Introduction

Saad, Lydia. (2025). Gallup. Americans' Ratings of U.S. Professions Historically Low

Retrieved from: https://news.gallup.com/poll/655106/americans-ratings-professions-stay-historically-low.aspx#:~:text=Nurses%20have%20earned%20the%20highest,attacks%20on%20the%20Twin%20Towers.

Lynaugh, J. (1989). Riding the yo-yo: The worth and work of nursing in the 20th century. Transactions and Studies of the College of Physicians of Philadelphia.11(ser. 5), Pgs. 201-217.

Reverby, S. (1987). Ordered to care. The dilemma of American nursing. Cambridge: Cambridge University Press

Goldmark. J. (1984). Nursing and nursing education in the United States. (Reprint ed.) New York: Garland Publishing Co. (original work published by The Macmillan Co., New York, 1923).

Burgess, M.A. (Ed.). (1984). Nurses, patients, and pocketbooks. (Reprint ed.) New York: Garland Publishing Co. (Original published by the Committee on the Grading of Nursing Schools, New York, 1928).

Falk, I.S., Rufus Rorem, C., & Ring, R. (1933). The Costs of Medical Care. Chicago: University of Chicago Press. Retrieved from: https://archive.org/details/dli.ministry.11553/page/n21/mode/2up

Egenes KJ. (n.d.). History of Nursing. Retrieved from: http://www.jblearning.com/samples/0763752258/52258_CH01_Roux.pdf.

McIver, P. (1942). Registered nurses in the U.S.A. American Journal of Nursing, 42, Pgs. 769-773.

Reverby, S. (1983). 'Something besides waiting": The politics of private duty reform in the depression. In E. C. Lagerman (Ed.), Nursing history, new perspectives, new possibilities Pgs. 133-156. New York: Teachers College Press.

United States Department of Labor (1948). Economic status of registered professional nurses, 1946-47 Bureau of Labor Statistics. Prepared for Ewan Clague, Commissioner

Willis D, Maples PG, Britton K. (2013). The Nurse Practice Act. Retrieved from: http://www.rochestergeneral.org/rochester-general-hospital/about-us/rochester-medical-museum-and-archives/online-exhibits/the-nursing-practice-act-the-armstrong-act-of-1903/

Alghamdi, M. G. (2016). Nursing Workload: Aconcept analysis. Journal of Nursing Management, 24 (4), Pgs. 449-457.

Habasevich, B. (2012). Defining acuity. [Blog post] June 26. Retrieved from:

http://www.mediware.com/rehabilitation/blog/item/defining-acuity/

NSI (2024). National Health Care Retention & RN Staffing Report. Retrieved from: https://nsinursingsolutions.com/Library.php

Edmonson, C. Zelonka, C. (2019). Our Own Worst Enemies: The Nurse Bullying Epidemic. Nursing Administration Quarterly 43(3): Pgs. 274-279, July/September 2019.

Hoover, M., Mahoney, K., Lucy, I. (2024). Data deep dive: A national nursing crisis. U.S. Chamber of Commerce Publication. Retrieved from: https://www.uschamber.com/workforce/nursing-workforce-data-center-a-national-nursing-crisis

AACN (2024). American Association of Colleges of Nursing. Nursing Workforce Fact Sheet Retrieved from: https://www.aacnnursing.org/news-data/fact-sheets/nursing-workforce-fact-sheet

Nightingale 1- Culture

ANA. (2013). Why Nurses Quit and Leave the Profession. Retrieved from:

https://www.nursingworld.org/content-hub/resources/nursing-leadership/why-nurses-quit/

Connors R. and Smith T., (2011). Change the Culture Change the Game, Penguin Group Inc., New York. Pg. 12.

Stone, D., Heen, S. (2014). Thanks for the feedback: The science and art of receiving feedback well. Pgs.17-20.

Grenny, J., Patterson, K., McMillan, R., Switzler, A., Gregory, E. (2021). Crucial conversations: Tools for talking when stakes are high (3rd ed.). McGraw Hill. Pg. 4, Pg. 144

McGovern, M. (2023). The problems with 'culture cliques' — and 5 ways to fix them. HRMorning. Retrieved from: https://www.hrmorning.com/articles/culture-cliques/

Ofei, A.M.A., Poku, C.A., Paarima, Y. (2023). Toxic leadership behaviour of nurse managers and turnover intentions: the mediating role of job satisfaction. BMC Nurs 22, Pg.374. Retrieved from:

https://doi.org/10.1186/s12912-023-01539-8

Goleman D. (1998). Working With Emotional Intelligence. New York: Bantam Books.

Kimura, H. (2003). Overcome toxic management. Nursing Management, 34(1), Pgs. 26-29.

Nightingale 2- Councils

CHCM (2023). Unlocking Success: Unit-based Council Ideas for Shared Governance in Hospitals; 37 (2): Pgs. 76-78. Pgs. 81-82 Retrieved from: doi:10.1177/1942602X211056371

Emily B., Brooklyn, C. (2022). Developing Tomorrow's Leaders Through Unit-Based Councils, Nurse Leader, Volume 20, Issue 6, Pgs. 565-568. Retrieved from: https://doi.org/10.1016/j.mnl.2022.08.002.

Nightingale 3- Coaching Precepting

Hardie, P., Murray, A., Jarvis, S. (2022). Experienced based co design: nursing preceptorship educational programme. Research Involvement and Engagement 8, 53. Pg. 3 Retrieved from: https://doi.org/10.1186/s40900-022-00385-3

Löfmark A., Thorkildsen K., Råholm M.B., Natvig G.K. (2012). Nursing students' satisfaction with supervision from preceptors and teachers during clinical practice. Nurse Education Practice 2012; 12. Pgs. 164– 169.

Benner, P., Tanner, C.A. and Chesla, A. (2009). Expertise in nursing practice: Caring, clinical judgment & ethics. Springer Publishing Company, New York.

Nightingale 5- Capabilities

AMN. (2024). survey of hospital nurse leaders. AMN Healthcare. Pg. 7.

Retrieved from: https://www.amnhealthcare.com/contentassets/6bc4f2d23e9d48f5aedd17b0a4f055ff/amn-survey-nurseleaders-2024-final.pdf

NSI. (2024). NSI national health care retention & RN staffing report. NSI Nursing Solutions. Retrieved from: https://www.nsinursingsolutions.com/documents/library/nsi_national_health_care_retention_report.pdf

Carroll, V. S. (2014). Transparency. The Journal of neuroscience nursing : journal of the American Association of Neuroscience Nurses, 46(1), Pg. 1. Retrieved from: https://doi.org/10.1097/JNN.0000000000000043

Apold, J. (2019). Leadership Rounding, listening and leading with purpose. Pg 7. Retrieved from chromeextension://efaidnbmnnnibpcajpcglclefindmkaj/https://www.leadingagemn.org/assets/docs/SCFS-LeadershipRounding-Oct19_(1).pdf

Schatz, B. (2022). The Huddle: A Daily Dose of Communication. NASN School Nurse. 37 (2): Pgs. 76-78. Retrieved from: doi:10.1177/1942602X211056371

Kahn, W. A. (1990). Psychological Conditions of Personal Engagement and Disengagement at Work. The Academy of Management Journal, 33(4), Pgs. 714–716. Retrieved from: https://doi.org/10.2307/256287

King, C., Bradley, L. A. (2023). PRC 2023 Nursing Engagement Report. Retrieved from: https://www.prcexcellence.com/wp-content/uploads/2019/PRC_Nursing_Engagement_Report/PRC-NurseReport-Final-031819-Secure.pdf

Gallup (2024). State of the global workplace: The voice of the world's employees. Retrieved from: https://www.gallup.com/workplace/349484/state-of-the-global-workplace.aspx

Miyata, A. , Arai, H. Suga, S. (2015). Nurse Managers Stress and Coping. *Open Journal of Nursing*, **5**, Pgs. 957-964. Retrieved from: doi: 10.4236/ojn.2015.511101

Goldsby, E., Goldsby, M., Neck, C. B., Neck, C. P. (2020). Under Pressure: Time Management, Self-Leadership, and the Nurse Manager. *Administrative Sciences.* 10 (3): Pg. 38. Retrieved from: https://doi.org/10.3390/admsci10030038

Kirman J. (2016). Behavioural interviewing as part of values-based recruitment for postgraduate community nursing programmes. Community practitioner : the journal of the Community Practitioners' & Health Visitors' Association, 89(9), Pgs. 42–47.

Sherman, R. O. (2019). The nurse leader coach: Become the boss no one wants to leave. Pg. 133, Pg.149

Frase-Blunt, M. (2004). Making exit interviews work. Society for Human Resource Management. Retrieved from: https://www.shrm.org/topics-tools/news/hr-magazine/making-exit-interviews-work

Cline, D., Curtin, K. Patricia A. Johnston P A., (2019). Professional Organization Membership The benefits of increasing nursing participation. Oncology Nursing Society (23) 5, Pg. 3. Retrieved from: chromeextension://efaidnbmnnnibpcajpcglclefindmkaj/https://www.ons.org/system/files/journal-article-pdfs/ProfessionOctober2019.pdf

Unit Champions

White, C. (2011). May 2011 Journal of Emergency Nursing 37(4): Pgs. 386- 387

Retrieved from: DOI:10.1016/j.jen.2011.04.009

Unit Council Images

Image from Eisenhower Medical Center. Retrieved from:

https://chcm.com/unit-based-council-ideas/ (2023)

Image from UC Davis Medical Center. Retrieved from:

https://health.ucdavis.edu/nurse/practicemodel/governance.html

www.ingramcontent.com/pod-product-compliance
Lightning Source LLC
LaVergne TN
LVHW050914210926
848482LV00012B/436